The Dress Doctor

by EDITH HEAD
and JANE KESNER ARDMORE

With Photographs

LITTLE, BROWN AND COMPANY Boston Toronto

All photographs courtesy of Paramount Pictures Corporation

Certain selections from this book appeared first in Good House-
keeping *in an article entitled "I Dress the World's Most
Glamorous Women."*

*Published simultaneously in Canada
by Little, Brown & Company (Canada) Limited*

PRINTED IN THE UNITED STATES OF AMERICA

Contents

Photographs appear between pages 112–113 and 136–137

The Dress Doctor

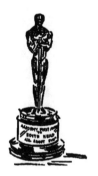

THE TIME: Today.

THE PLACE: The doctor's "operating room" at Paramount Studios, Hollywood — and unlike any other operating room in the world. Pale silver gray, this suite; very cool, very elegant, with silver-gray carpets, silver-gray walls, French Provincial furniture covered in silver leaf, the lights reflected in antiqued mirrors which illumine walls, doors and coffee table. Mirrored doors at the far end swing together during a fitting to leave doctor and patient alone under the merciless lights. Then the doors swing open, and the atmosphere is again that of the austere drawing room.

Little dressmaker forms from the Flea Market in Paris stand in beheaded grace on several tables surrounded by miniature antique sewing machines from every corner of the world. Sunlight, slanting through French windows, dances on the six dazzling golden "boys" — Academy Award Oscars, highest tribute of the motion picture industry to the skill of . . .

THE DOCTOR: EDITH HEAD, whose magic can transform any woman — make her appear fat or thin, rich or poor, old or young, ingenue or sophisticate — she who daily translates the most glamorous actresses in the world into the characters they play on screen.

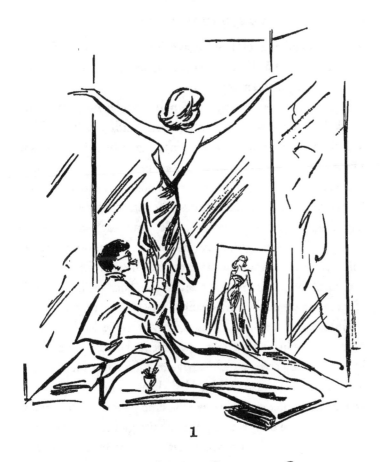

1

Today in My Fashion Clinic

AT THE CRACK of dawn, in comes Dietrich, looking — in sleek black leather pants and jacket — like all the fashion magazine covers rolled into one. (She and Roy Rogers are the only two living humans who should be allowed to wear such trousers!) You think of her as a night person? The bewitching *chanteuse* of Las Vegas? Symbol of glamour? You should see her at 6:30 A.M., without make-up, freshly scrubbed and crackling with energy.

I'm as hardened as anyone can be to glamour, stars, the whole Hollywood routine; but Dietrich is still a thrill, and her arrival heralds a stimulating, exciting, exhausting time. Queen Dietrich is — heaven help us — *the* perfectionist. No hook or eye, no seam is unimportant. It can take days and more days. Crews may falter, fitters faint, designers contemplate hara-kiri; Dietrich remains indefatigable, and each detail must be right. Once it's right, it can be better. She never raises her voice, she never grows impatient, but Dietrich fittings aren't over until the picture is; and a few weeks later she'll still think of some iota we might have changed. What's more, she knows.

Fashion is a language. Some know it, some learn it, some never will — like an instinct. I've spent the best years of my life with young actresses who arrive in ruffles, pinafores, fuzzy-headed and with diamond-buckled shoes. They listen, learn, and in short order not only have the chic pattern, they actually think they were born wearing little white gloves! But Dietrich was born knowing, and when we work together, it is less doctor and patient than two specialists in consultation on the character in hand.

"So, we begin," says Dietrich, and thumps down a fantastic piece of French luggage, leather and canvas. Out of it come a Thermos of coffee — for us; when she's working she needs no nourishment — books, scripts, an extra pair of shoes, and one of her famous tortes, a seven-layer cake she learned to make in Vienna. She wastes no motion. Before the triple mirrors in my gray operating room, she quickly peels down, revealing the most beautiful French lingerie I've ever seen, all white, just a touch of lace.

"I have been reading the script," she says in her slow, low voice. ". . . Have some coffee, Edith, it helps. We are going to have trouble with this woman?" She speaks of the woman in the glass, as if that were a third person she and I were discussing. "This woman is not going to be so easy."

And she is so right. The picture is *Witness for the Prosecution;* as a physician who can change anyone, through the medicine of dress, my task is to change Marlene from one of the smartest of women into just an average female: obliterate the Dietrich look, make her as little Dietrich as possible. The audience simply must not gasp when she walks into the scene. She must look like a middle-class woman in ready-made English winter clothes of about five years ago — not sophisticated, certainly not glamorous.

To make our task more difficult, the script calls for *two tailored suits.* (If you want the most elegant female in the world, you put Dietrich in a tailored suit — the plainer the suit, the more elegant she) — and *one gaudy costume* for the flashback, where she will play a London streetwalker. . . . Just three changes, but these three call for more ingenuity than all the lovely clothes for *Funny Face,* more effort than all the costumes for *The Ten Commandments.*

The diagnosis starts . . . not with measurements. We have Dietrich's measurements from *A Foreign Affair* (1948), and her figure doesn't vary although she eats like a truck horse. We start with fabrics. Lined up across the room are bolts and bolts of materials. Fitters haul each bolt so I can drape the fabrics across her famous chassis. On the bolt this brown wool looks coarse enough, but draped on her it looks . . .

"As if I were going to Pavillon for lunch!" says Marlene. "It's too *beautiful*."

We try a rough, bulky tweed; this is so wrong it becomes a caricature no one would believe. There's a fine line between clothes that will help her become the character and clothes that are a clumsy disguise. Marlene understands this; she understands too — as Anna Magnani understands, as Shirley Booth understands, and Katharine Hepburn — the difference between fashion and costume. Fashion is the current mode; it enables each woman to dramatize herself for the moment. Costume is the province of the theatrical designer, clothes which can help an actress become the character demanded by the script.

"The producer and the director are worried, Marlene; they want you to look like a *hausfrau*. The question is, what does a *hausfrau* look like? Homesy? Ginghamy? Provincial? Dowdy?"

"Why don't they ask me?" laughs Dietrich. "I *was* one!" She shakes her head, shakes the hair she wears shoulder-long, as she did ten years ago. "I was not dowdy."

"You were an actress first, a *hausfrau* second."

We find a tweed that looks pretty good. Dietrich goes for cups, pours coffee for everyone. While we sip, she starts trying some of the skirt patterns I've cut. Half of what's made the Dietrich look is the carriage, the long slim legs; so this time I try swinging the skirt out, away from the body.

"Good," she says, walking up and down in medium-heeled English walking shoes, holding the skirt pattern. "For the flashback, Edith, she should have some platform shoes with ankle straps, very hussy, red."

One of the crew goes to Wardrobe to hunt for red platforms while Marlene tries blouses, slowly, methodically buttoning every button of every blouse. *Forty* blouses.

"There are hats downstairs in the car," she says, "I made the rounds of the studios borrowing hats." Two of my girls go downstairs, come back staggering under the load of berets, cloches, sailors.

"No red platform shoes in Miss Dietrich's size," comes word from the shoe section. We call MGM, Western Costume, Warners', Columbia. No luck. . . . "It looks as if we may have to find something else."

"We will find *them*," she says quietly. "Red, with platforms and ankle straps, very hussy. Tomorrow, Edith, you and I will go downtown early, to Main Street, to Spring Street; we'll wear scarfs over our heads, hm? and find funny shoes and hats with character. Poor Billie, you look so tired — let me make more coffee." She starts for the hot plate wearing a battered cloche that makes her look (shrugging her shoulders) exactly like Dietrich! We drink gallons of coffee and she tries on hats, hats, hats.

I'm reminded of the time we first met, years and years ago,

in the interests of a white feather hat. Marlene was a great star then and I was a pencil pusher, Travis Banton's sketch artist and assistant; the only actors I ever met were the maids, the grandmothers, or the heroines of "B" westerns. A very important hat of filmy, gossamer white feathers had been made for Dietrich; the scene was to be shot the next morning; Travis had left the lot for another fitting. At four in the afternoon, in walked Dietrich with her hands full of feathers. The hat could be better, she thought, and she spent the night *making* it better — the first do-it-yourselfer I'd met in Hollywood.

She was terribly engrossed in the feathers that night, yet somehow, before morning, she'd become interested in me too. People don't usually get to know me easily, I'm not a great giver-outer; habitually, I keep my problems to myself; and most stars would scarcely have been aware of a sketch artist. But Miss Dietrich discovered that I wasn't terribly happy, that I was worried about my career (if you could call it that at the time), that I had a horrible feeling I was going to be stuck forever designing duds for horse operas.

"We must have your horoscope cast!" she declared, jotting down the date of my birth. "You have not had your horoscope?" In nothing flat, I received my horoscope from her astrologer.

BETTER TIMES ARE COMING, it said.

I had a warm feeling for Marlene Dietrich from that day, a growing admiration, too, for her sense of perfection. Travis once designed a priceless gown for her, an evening sheath beaded solidly in pearls, rubies and diamonds — semiprecious.

Out in the workroom, I watched her patiently move one diamond on that dress fifty times until it came at last to rest in the place where its effect was maximum.

The clincher came on an evening when I was sent to her home to help her dress for a costume ball. She was going as Leda in a bit of chiffon with the Swan draped over her shoulder. The Swan was part of the costume; it had to be arranged so that it leaned, gazing into her eyes. As I brought the swan's head into position, Dietrich started.

"He's all wrong!" she cried. "Who ever heard of a *blue-eyed* swan?"

From that moment, she was my girl, and I dreamed of the day when I would design for her a magnificent, high-fashion wardrobe. So what happened? In *A Foreign Affair* she played herself, a woman entertaining the troops, and had to wear a raincoat, an old dressing gown and a battered suit. The script did call for a shimmering evening gown, but she wore one she'd actually worn entertaining behind the front lines. Now I have her for *Witness for the Prosecution* and am dressing her down to character-size. It's a blow, because she's certainly the most beautiful of women, the model every designer would most like to dress; and because — we're friends. In a business where friendships are often transient and you learn to guard yourself to keep from getting hurt, Marlene is that rare person you can trust. This is no perennial orchid, drinking champagne in bed; this is an energetic woman with the common touch. She likes cooking, she likes sewing, she likes children and grandchildren, she likes people. In her French lingerie and a mannish hat, she has just stopped to show us pictures of her grandchildren, her daughter, her son-in-law.

Now she slips into the first of a pile of jackets, sent in from Wardrobe. Any reasonable jacket molds to her and becomes stylish; what we'll have to do is make the lapels a little too large and a little too low, strike a length in-between, neither short and boxy nor long and slim. . . . I have a pattern cut, hold it to her; and there she is — Dior's darling, looking reasonably everyday.

A frantic point of red light flashes on my phone. Urgent. It's the production manager on the *Houseboat* set. I'm to come at once: Sophia Loren's gold dress has just turned Cary Grant — the whole front of him — solid gold.

Marlene cheerfully waves me away. "Tomorrow I will pick you up at eight; we'll go to Spring street . . ." She should be exhausted, she should look like a wreck. She looks exactly as she did when she arrived. I slip into flat-heeled shoes, wish I had time to smooth my own hair, and hurry down the stairs.

Like everyone else at Paramount, I have a bicycle. Unlike anyone else, I've never learned to ride it. There's nothing to do but trot to Stage 16, a sleeper-jump away.

On the set — pandemonium, a buzz of laughter, a state of shock; everyone is upset except Sophia, and she is laughing the deep, infectious laugh that ripples her gold dress. Every time she glances at Cary Grant, she laughs again. They have been dancing and he looks a little like Sir Galahad in shining armor. Let me explain that in the script another woman has given Sophia the flamboyant dress (gold, smothered in gold roses and trimmed with red ribbon) in the hope that it will look cheap and gaudy and repel Mr. Grant. In an unexpected way, it has done just that. The dress is of jersey impregnated with 14-karat gold, something I've never used before, and against Cary's impeccable English dinner clothes it has achieved an all but gold-plate.

I send at once to the studio paintshop for a strange dress medicine: lacquer and a spray gun to spray Miss Loren, it's such an instant drying lacquer, she needn't even disrobe. Cary Grant has meanwhile been carefully dusted off; and now, hold her tight as he will, the gold stays put!

After the take, Sophia walks over to her husband, Carlo Ponti, who has just come on the set. "You think this is a dress," she says. "It is not. I am like an Oscar, sprayed on."

With the exception of this gold dress, Sophia wears beautiful modern clothes for the first time on the screen in *House-boat*. Originally, she was to have been an American girl; and when I first went to see her, I came bearing sketches of a girl in blue jeans, sweatshirts, the clothes an American girl would wear on such a boat. Miss Loren couldn't have been more charming — or more horrified.

"I do not wear blue jeans," she said in her beautiful English.

I took a good look at the clothes she does wear: very high-fashion, very elegant: dress, shoes, jewelry by top Italian designers. She is the exact antithesis of the Italian character roles she has played on screen, the exact antithesis of the earthy, sexy type I'd expected. We expect Italian, French and

Spanish girls to be highly emotional, slightly volcanic and of the earth earthy. Sophia is the most poised person with whom I've ever worked, thoroughly organized, dignified and slightly formal. She wasn't about to call me "Edith," at least in the first five minutes. And I liked it. She told me her preference in clothes, soft colors: beiges, pale mauve, soft olive-green (her colors complement her eyes, which are soft green, like a tiger's); no frills, no adornment, the plainer the better. She is quite right. The closer she resembles a statue, the better she looks and the better-proportioned her clothes appear.

So I retreated gracefully, went to the director and producer and suggested we change the American girl on a houseboat to an Italian girl on a houseboat. "There's nothing wrong with her figure," I explained, "but she isn't the cowboy type." Since then, Sophia and I have gotten on tremendously. She wastes no time, no energy, she uses no word whiskers (no "Well — uh . . ." or "But I'm not — uh sure — uh . . ."), and I like her, respect her; I'm even learning to speak Italian!

"*L'attendo alle quatro* [I expect you at four this afternoon]," I remind her. We must fit one of her somber costumes for "The Black Orchid," also her handsome Academy Award dress.

"I will be there," she says solemnly (and it will be four sharp, you can count on that), turning away to dance once again, this time for the close-up, with Cary Grant.

I hurry back to my Clinic. It's almost 12:30. Kim Novak is due for a fitting for *Vertigo;* we will have lunch sent in. . . . Take a deep breath. It's been a strenuous morning, and I'm not looking forward to Kim because I have to fit her in something she's not going to like — a gray tailored suit. As she told me at our first meeting, "I'll wear anything — so long as it isn't a suit; any color — so long as it isn't gray." Then she looked at me with those big brown eyes while I explained the story point.

This girl must look as if she's just drifted out of the San Francisco fog. She is walking, driving a car and walking in San Francisco, so it can't be a gray chiffon *peignoir*. In this city everyone wears suits, and this girl is a rather withdrawn, self-contained, tailored type. Mr. Hitchcock has already shot the location; he wants the girl to seem a very part of the fog; his script calls for, specifically, a *gray tailored suit*. Also, Mr. Hitchcock has in him a streak of Gibraltar.

"If it has to be a suit," Kim said, "I like *purple* suits, or *white* suits. Naturally, I want to do what Mr. Hitchcock wants, but . . ."

So today we're fitting the gray suit. In a case like this, you don't mention any anesthetic, you just use one. The anesthetic will be a black satin gown and black satin coat lined with emerald green which she'll wear in the restaurant scene. Kim plays two different people in this picture — one a slightly neurotic woman with taste and money, the other a vital girl who loves dancing, is full of the *joie de vivre*. Every line of monotone tailleur can help define the first woman, every bright color will help convey the second. Neither of the characters is the real Kim.

Off screen, this is a very pretty young woman who looks

like an actress. She has much more warmth and personality than on screen, and she hasn't been in this business long enough to lose any of her enthusiasm; she's changeable, mercurial, not a bit blasé! Today she's wearing her favorite lavender (she likes any color, so long as it's purple, violet or lavender), lavender slacks and a purple sweater. With her is her companion, Luddy Lane, and I'm asking them what they want from the commissary when Kim starts waving a basket under my nose, they've just come from the Farmers' Market and they've brought lunch with them.

"Have some Rabbit's Delight," says Kim, producing cucumbers, lettuce, carrots and tomatoes, and relishing the piece of tomato she pops into her mouth as someone else would relish candy. "Good for your nerves, Edith — you should eat lots of carrots!" We each have paper napkins and a lap full of vegetables.

When we have consumed the greenery, the "operation" gets under way; and working with every star is major, believe me. There has never been an actress with whom it is easy to work. Comedian or tragedian, five years old or seventy-five, each of them really thinks she knows more than I do about her hipline, her bustline and her neckline. A dress doctor without diplomacy — or worse, without a flair for psychoanalysis — is sunk. So I show Kim a raft of handsome suit sketches and swatches of the most beautiful sheer wool fabrics you've ever seen: cold grays, warm grays, pink grays, blue grays, slate grays. . . . Grays can be very lovely, this misty one, for example, looks as if the sun were coming through.

"Where did you find that?" Kim says. "It's beautiful! I don't mind wearing *that* gray at all."

It's material I'd found in London, the very color of a London fog. Albert, the tailor, comes in to fit the suit pattern — a man who has fitted every star in the business. I've worked with him for twenty years. He is a tall, blond German. Kim looks up at him and says, "Albert, do you mind? Let me see if the suit will work." And she puts her arms on his shoulders as she'll put her arms on tall Jimmy Stewart's shoulders in the actual scene. Albert is laughing, flustered, completely captivated by her.

Then we fit the black satin. This is more Kim's style. She isn't actually a suit girl, she's a lovely female animal with the walk and the figure that makes an evening gown seductive. This is how she likes to look on the screen, how she likes to feel — beautiful.

What a contrast to my next patient, Shirley Booth, to whom (as an actress) clothes are just the means of projecting a part. I've had Shirley in *Come Back Little Sheba, About Mrs. Leslie,* and now *The Matchmaker.* She never analyzes clothes as becoming or unbecoming, good, bad or indifferent, all she asks is, "What will they do for the scene?" (Remember the dowdy, sleazy bathrobe in *Sheba?*)

Well, for *The Matchmaker* I tried to gild the lily a bit, and for the big dinner scene I did a dress with a few spangles and a little feather boa, a rose for her hair. How she laughed. "I look good enough to be Lillian Russell at Delmonico's," she said, and promptly started switching, the skirt of one dress to the top of another, little bits and pieces. "Remember," she said, "I'm the kind of woman who makes her own clothes; I would have a bit of an old drape, a scrap of tablecloth, patchwork." So she scrambled my costumes to make them more homemade, to achieve the humorous effect she felt she must have for the character, an effect I couldn't possibly know from reading the script.

When the call comes from the set that Shirley Booth wants to see me at once, I wonder if some of Shirley's patchwork has come apart? I leave Kim finishing up with the fitters and hurry to *The Matchmaker* set. Shirley is sitting in a hopeless jumble of finery in her dressing room; she isn't working in the current scene.

"Edith, you always see me in rags and patches," laughs Shirley. "I want you to see how I *can* look!" And she slips a color transparency into a small viewer. There in the viewer is a stunning woman, her hair a rich red-gold, her dress, amber. When she was in Europe a few months ago, she explains, she had some wonderful clothes made. If you think of her as a woman in an old bathrobe or a housedress, clothes that look as if they were her last refuge, you should see her in the high fashion she wears: shades of amber, strange hyacinth blues, gray-greens, the color magic of her personal wardrobe. These transparencies are beautiful; and as I view them, her two white poodles, Grazie ("Thank You") and Prego ("You're Welcome") sit up on their respective chairs as if it were indeed a fashion show. The poodles, both girls, hate each other,

but they're the best-behaved dogs who've ever invaded my
fitting room, and they adore fashion as Shirley does.

"Miss Booth!" They're calling her for a scene now, and
she bustles away, no longer the chic Shirley Booth, but Mrs.
Levi in gay, awful clothes, her mind on the business of mat-
rimony.

I stop by the set of *Teacher's Pet* to check with Clark Cable
— there's a scene coming up in which Doris Day will wear
a sharp gray flannel suit and it's important that he not wear
a gray flannel suit. I also want to talk about what he will wear
in his next picture with Carroll Baker and Lilli Palmer.

Back to my Clinic. Waiting is the smart blocked-print
skirt Sophia will wear over her bathing suit. I try it on, over
my tweed suit. The effect is pretty funny. Sophia is 5'8, I'm
barely 5'1. Sophia has the measurements of a Venus de Milo,
I'm the approximate prototype of an ironing board; but I
have to see how a dress works, how it moves, walks, sits. I
try everything on myself. This tie-on overskirt is a direct
decendant of the famous Lamour sarong. It works, even over
my tweeds. I try on her black mourning dress and then
the glimmering sheath of pearl silk shot with gold Sophia will
wear for the Academy Awards.

When I've taken this back to the workroom for a few added
darts, I'm startled, coming into my office, to see a man in work
clothes and heavy shoes; it would seem he's fixing the radiator,
his feet in the air. He rolls over, jumps nimbly to his feet
and it's — Sophia Loren! Her afternoon fitting has cut her
gym time, so . . .

"I exercise every day, twenty minutes at least," she explains. "Look, I will show you how."

We call in my secretary, Cathryn, my sketch artist, Grace, and have an impromptu gym class; but Sophia's the only one of us who can do these exercises; Yul Brynner *couldn't*. She laughs at us and that's enchanting, because she laughs so seldom.

The phone rings. Deborah Kerr, wanting to talk about a benefit at which she's appearing. . . . WHAT SHOULD SHE WEAR? . . . Sophia is standing before the mirrors in her pearl sheath. She wonders about furs: WHAT SHOULD SHE WEAR? . . . Zsa Zsa Gabor pokes her wild blond head in: DAHLING, WHAT SHOULD I WEAR? . . . The phone again. My boss, to tell me I'm being loaned to Hecht-Hill Lancaster. It's an emergency. Rita Hayworth is to start *Separate Tables* in a week, I'll have two days to design the high-fashion modes: WHAT SHOULD MISS HAYWORTH WEAR?

Cathryn brings in a pile of letters and puts them in the center of my desk. They're from all over the country — I end my day with them every day — from women who want to know: WHAT SHOULD THEY WEAR? To a wedding, a tea, a P.T.A. meeting: WHAT SHOULD THEY WEAR?

Smile at the title "Dress Doctor," but clothes are a practical therapy, and a woman's happiness — her outlook on life, her ability to meet the terrible competition in love and in war, in business and before the eagle eye of her sisters — can be decided by WHAT SHE WEARS. The way you dress affects you;

it also affects the people around you. Every woman has weapons. One of them is color: color not only can change the way a woman looks, it can change the way she feels, the way she thinks.

There should be no badly dressed American women, because today clothes are available at any price range, from a few to a thousand dollars. They are badly dressed because there have been no rules. A woman who wouldn't think of essaying food preparation without recipes from a good cookbook goes groping for clothes with no mother to guide her. One hundred years ago, every woman wore a hoopskirt, she had no choice; seventy-five years ago, every woman wore a bustle. Today, a woman can look any way she wishes — if she knows how, if there is someone to help her. Every woman is a ham actress at heart; she can be transformed to glamour as we transform the professional actresses to glamour, day after day throughout the years.

It's to Mrs. Average American this book is dedicated. She has been in my mind, my thoughts and experiments ever since I first hung out my shingle.

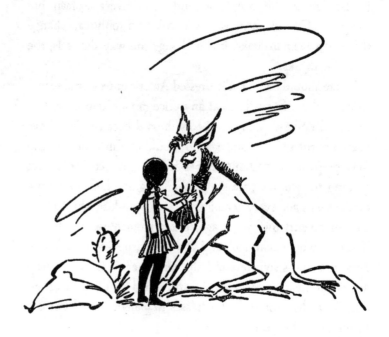

2

The Same Doctor—The First Patients

THE HOUSE WAS of unpainted wood with a porch on three sides, a slanted tar-paper roof, a jutting stovepipe, and as far as you could see — north, east, south and west — nothing to break the monotony, just this house sitting on the stony desert floor, not a tree or a shrub, not a blade of grass. And sitting on the porch, alone in the glaring sun, a small dark-eyed child with black hair in plaits, a starched Peter Thomson dress, long black cotton stockings. I remember it all acutely. It was our house and I was that child.

My stepfather was a mining engineer, and of all the mining camps we lived in, this is the one I remember best, four miles out of a metropolis called Searchlight, Nevada. A prospector, Fred Colton, had drifted into this area around the turn of the century and thought it a likely spot for a gold mine. His partner told him he'd need a searchlight to find anything there, so Searchlight it became, population about five hundred. I hated the loneliness of the desert, dreamed of cities, of play-mates, of sounds, of people next door; but I loved it, too — the cactus and greasewood that sprawled on the desert floor, the tiny yellow flowers in spring. Greasewood is pliable; I'd bend it into little figures with arms and legs and stick them in the sand. Sometimes I'd find mannequins already formed and growing, just waiting for hats of desert flowers. Lots of tiny people standing about in the sand, talking to each other; beside them, I'd decorate a greasewood bush with bits of sparkling tin foil.

Mother would call me to come back, come back; she didn't like me to wander away from the house because of snakes. There were rattlesnakes, scorpions and tarantulas — that's why everyone wore boots. It's why we looked under the beds every night, too. Once mother did find me asleep on the woodpile and, right beside me, coiled up in the sun and sound asleep, a giant rattler. I had no fear. My theory was *Let them alone, they'll let you alone,* and it worked pretty well.

I loved animals; they were my best friends. Every afternoon of the world you'd find us out behind the kitchen door
in the shade having a tea party. I used a cardboard packing
box for a table; the tea cloth was one of mother's red-checked
linen towels; the dishes were doll-size Haviland, and there was
a suitable supply of dainty sandwiches and cambric tea. But
what made the tea parties as mad as any attended by Alice
in Wonderland were my guests and their getups: my black
cat, Tom, and my white dog, Dina, nicely dressed in doll
clothes; a horned toad, a jackrabbit, a burro or two, all gussied
up in feathers and ribbons, with necklaces of crepe paper.
Burros wandered around the camp at will, once in a while
one wandered into our kitchen and mother would have hys-
terics; but I found them very friendly. There were a couple
tame enough to ride, and I could persuade them, with bribes of
scraps, to let me tie ribbons about their middles and decorate
their heads with scarves, ribbons or lace. "Mr. So and So"
and "Mrs. So and So," I called them. And if they seemed stubborn about their "fittings," that was only because at the time
I'd never met an actress.

Horned toads I'd find lying still on the sand, so nearly
desert-color you might step on them. They were only slightly
reluctant to be dressed for company tea. I'd always have
scraps of meat and bits of lettuce and chicken feed for the
animals, and we'd sit on the clean white sand while I carried
on the conversations, all of us floating in the warm, fruity
scent of tarts, the yeasty smell of bread swelling in mother's
kitchen.

My greatest treasure was my stock bag of scraps, most treasured of the scraps the old kid gloves, some of them opera-length, which were divine for upholstering furniture. Remember how Paulette Goddard used to carry around a cigar box filled with her priceless jewels? Well, cigar boxes meant little sofas to me; I'd upholster them elaborately in white kid and thumb tacks; they were just the right size for my toads. Four wooden boxes formed my doll house; in it I'd sit toads and an occasional doll.

My other great treasure was a collection of whisky bottles. This was a wide-open town; all along the road I'd find empty liquor bottles, some of them tinted by the sun. I stashed them under the house or hid them out back, and on a warm day I'd line them up in the sun in beautiful array. But there were days of violent wind too, when you shivered dressing beside the wood stove in the kitchen, when there was nothing to do but stay indoors. Then my mother would play with me. We played parchesi and, on the smooth linoleum floor of the kitchen, she taught me to play jacks: "Cows over the fence" . . . "Pigs in a poke" . . . Long after, when I first came to Paramount, I used to play jacks in a back fitting room with another designer, Milo Anderson. He was working for Mr. de Mille, but Mr. de Mille was on location and we were in a temporary lull when Travis Banton had nothing for me to do; so we'd rush in to work at the studio and promptly at 9 A.M. start playing jacks. Over the years with Mother, I'd developed into a championship player; jacks are my best sport.

My mother was a fantastic woman, now that I look back.

She was small, with black hair, blue eyes and fair coloring;
she loved everything nice, everything dainty. Yet she adapted
to mining camps and never seemed to mind at all! Everybody
adapted to life in Searchlight and seemed to enjoy it — I
could barely forgive them. (And whether I was adjusted
never occurred to anyone, least of all to me.) Because Mother
liked things nice, dreary dreadful place that this was, she
always had white organdy curtains at the windows, ruffled;
she used her sterling silver every day and her Haviland china.
"You never know when you'll be taken," she said; and she
made our kitchen a gay one, the sun pouring over the red-
and-white-checked or blue-and-white-checked tablecloths, on
Sunday a white one. I knew it was Sunday because of the
white cloth and because Old Tom came to Sunday dinner.

He was an aged prospector who'd been around Searchlight
forever. Mother asked him to dinner because he had no
one. When she served him her wonderful hot apple pie,
he'd slather it with butter, and that made her furious; but
she always asked him the next Sunday again, and he was
with us on Christmas when we had open house and my stepfather, who was superintendent, played host to the miners
and their families. Our house was like a railroad station on
Christmas; there were oranges and gilded nuts for us children (a special treat sent from Los Angeles), whisky and
boxes of cigars for the miners. Mother'd make the men step
outside to smoke so as not to smell up her white organdy
curtains.

Old Tom went with us on picnics, too. We'd hitch up big

fat Charlie and we'd go out under the joshua trees. Everyone from the mine and everyone from the town would be
there: the doctor, the saloon keeper, the mine owners, everyone came and cooked. There were whole steers sizzling in
pits, and kegs of beer; Old Tom would get a little drunk and
he'd fall asleep. Then Old Tom died one day and left *everything* to my mother. There was a big write-up about it in
the paper and every charity in the state applied to mother
for a donation. (Of course the paper had failed to say how
much he'd left. Old Tom's *everything* was one hundred and
fifty dollars.)

From time to time, as a special treat, my stepfather would
take me down into the mine itself. We'd ride in an elevator
with no sides, down level after level in the cold dark. It was
fascinating, but I was glad to get back up into the sunlight,
to the flat endless wasteland and the chickens pecking away
at the gravel. I always thought those chickens pretty stupid.

The one real break in monotony was going to town. We'd
drive down the main street, past the iron corrugated buildings
to Hinke and Scott's general merchandise store, where you
could buy anything: coal, oil, crayons and any meat that had
been hauled in from Manvel, twenty-eight miles away on the
branch railroad that came from Santa Fe (we ate little meat,
mostly chicken, cottontail, quail and game). Down the main
street we went, past the buildings of corrugated iron — only
the jail was a tent. I guess we didn't have much crime in
Searchlight. My stepfather said mostly it was just crooked

gamblers, and they were sent on their way with a lunchbox and a canteen of water — which was not bad, he said, considering as how a fifty-gallon barrel of drinking water cost five dollars.

While my parents shopped, they dropped me off at the doctor's to play with his two little girls, Marjorie and her younger sister Helène. They were my only friends and I loved them madly, especially Marjorie, who was my age. They were blondes with curly hair and blue eyes, and I hated them madly, too, because I'd have given anything in the world for curly hair *any* color. We used to play charades and amateur theatricals, and I always assigned myself the part of the boy or the mother; I wasn't about to compete with two curly-headed blondes!

I dressed *them* up in the best ribbons, feathers and kid gloves from my stock bag. Because my stock bag went right with me to town, the doctor's wife and all the other ladies saved their scraps of material for me. I went from house to house collecting loot.

But the visits to town were few and far between and time passed slowly. The only security I seemed to have were my animal friends, and even the fairy tales I dreamed had animals as their characters. When the summer grew hot, I left Searchlight for another world, I went to visit my own father, who lived in El Paso, a slender man with brown, thinking eyes and a mustache. They all had mustaches, my father, my stepfather and Old Tom (my father patted his with a napkin after eating, just so); the difference was my father wore his

hair parted in the center and a bow tie, and he looked like a
poet — at least he looked as I thought a poet would look. He
was a fine Latin scholar, my father, a man who read a great
deal.

Often we would cross the border into Mexico and wander
up and down the streets of Juárez. I liked that. Everything
was gay and colorful; I loved the way the Mexican women
dressed. I still do. Any time I'm assigned a picture of any
period that deals with Latin America it's just like coming
home — I know it by heart; it's the one country I don't have
to research.

My first brush with the real world of fashion was when
my parents took me to New York. I must have been eight,
and I'll never forget Mother taking me shopping — buying
me a blue serge Peter Thomson dress with a high neck and
elbow-length sleeves; it was definitely my entrée into the
haut monde. In my new bib and tucker, we went to dinner
at an elegant restaurant, mother wore a dinner hat, and we
ate lobster! It came on a platter garnished with two porcelain
baby lobsters; I wanted to take one of them home with me.
At the Waldorf-Astoria Hotel, where we stopped, I had my
first real bath in a real bathtub. Instead of sitting, knees up,
in the old galvanized tub beside the kitchen stove, here I was
floating in splendor, to music from the hotel's roof garden.
The trip to New York had an unhappy dénouement — I was
fitted for glasses! It was the end of the world. I'd never
considered myself the Shirley Temple of Searchlight; as a

matter of fact, I was pretty negative about my possibilities, and glasses weren't going to add to my charm. So I never wore them (which is probably why I'm so near-sighted now).

With glasses I would certainly never have achieved my one moment of glamour — as Rosebud at the Valentine party! All the children were to be flowers, and at the crucial moment I took over and dictated who was to be the Daisy, who the Violet and who the Lily; I personally, said I, would be the Rosebud. I was, too, in pink Dennison crepe paper, my hair in perfect *curls*, achieved by the fairly arduous routine of wetting the hair, tying it on rags, and sleeping on the lumps till morning. The very reason for rushing madly into the occasion, I'm sure, was because it offered a chance for the curls, which usually were restricted to Christmas, July 4, May Day and my birthday.

The Valentine Day party was my first production, and my friend Marjorie, the doctor's daughter, recalls that I was quite a tartar, every crepe-paper costume was my responsibility. Not that I dreamed of being a dress designer. I'd never even heard of one; it looked more likely that I'd end up a hairdresser, at least mother thought so, as she watched the pains with which I made wigs and mustaches for my Easter eggs. I had no idea of being anything.

But when the time came for high school and we came to Los Angeles (I was twelve years old then), my inertia disappeared. I *had* to be something, and I started on a frenzied series of potential careers. The doctor's family was also living in Los Angeles, and Marjorie was taking music lessons from the great Olga Steeb; I decided that I would become a "great" concert pianist. We were living in an apartment house where there was a piano in the recreation room for practice, and mother sent me to Olga Steeb. She took only the talented, incidentally, and turned out some very fine musicians. After a valiant effort on both our parts, she sent a letter to mother to the effect that my lessons were a waste of time and money, I had no musical talent whatsoever.

I decided to become a "great" gymnast instead. Our apartment house was the Zelda Apartments, at Fourth and Grand; at the bottom of the hill was the YWCA. I enrolled for every class they had to offer. The classes were primarily for teachers and for women trying to lose weight, and here I was, a thirteen-year-old high school girl, very small for my age, in a middy blouse and bloomers. I lifted the bars, did calisthenics, trapeze work, played tennis and volleyball, swam like a channel aspirant for about a year. There were no other girls my age with whom to become friends; I grew tired of overstuffed women and their bulges (to this day an overweight actress brings them to mind); I grew bored with the idea of being a lady gymnast. Too, I was developing some very peculiar muscles.

I was probably the strongest girl in L. A. High, and I didn't know what to do with myself. I never had to work hard at studies because I have a photographic memory. To prepare for an exam, all I had to do was read the material. Of course, two weeks later it was all gone, but by that time I'd passed the exams. Math I never did get through, but by taking lots of

Latin, I compensated for that; and I played Aeneas in our play, *Dido, Regina Carthaginis.* (Not because I was popular but because everyone else was too lazy to learn that many lines.)

My parents had moved to the tungsten mine near Atolia now; I was living with mother's oldest friend, "Aunt" Mittie Morgan, on Sunset Place. Ducks became my hobby and I'm probably responsible today for all the ducks in Westlake Park. My entire allowance went for fertile duck eggs. I bought them at a pet shop, brought them home and turned them over to my mother duck. When the mother duck was *in absentia* (the neighbors sometimes complained), a hotwater bottle had to do. I must have raised two, three hundred ducks, I don't know how Aunt Mittie stood them.

My other mad passion was the movies. The biggest theater in town was the old Million Dollar Theater on Third Street; for a while I all but lived there. It was something to *do*. It was almost a relief, when summer came, to go out to Atolia in Death Valley, where the temperature was 116 on a cool day. The Fourth of July occasioned a holiday and the miners would go on a three-day binge of excitement. They'd have a rodeo, auto races, horse races and the grand climax — a big dance contest.

The summer before I went to college, I won the silver loving cup in the dance contest. Of course, there wasn't much competition, all the young people left Atolia in the summer to get away from the heat and I was the only girl in camp! I wore a dress of pale blue tulle and silver lamé (I loathe blue and hate lamé); I had a very gay young man as partner, a college student from Colorado who was studying metallurgy; and in all the heat we danced to a fare-thee-well. My loving cup was three feet high, later it turned coal-black.

At the University of California, I crept back into my shell. I put on the glasses I'd never worn before and wore them ceaselessly. I was not going to be an international beauty or a college belle, and on a campus as big and confusing as this I decided I'd better see where I was going. I think they became a protective coloration from the beginning, so effective that I never had any sense of being a part of the campus at all: I was a spectator. Only once did I ever take a leap into student activities, I went out for *rowing*. I'd never rowed before, my hands blistered even through gloves, my coordination was hilarious, and of course I was half as big as anyone else on the team; but I kept with it until I discovered that by the time I'd get back from Oakland, where we practiced, to the dorm at Berkeley, dinner was all over. My athletic career was not worth doing without dinner. I retired.

The one important thing that happened during my college years was the summers away from college. My father's close friends, Frank and Mabelle Spencer, invited me to visit them at the Grand Canyon. Frank Spencer was in charge of the Hopi House and the fabulous collection of Indian costumes and art. I fell in love with the Indians, their primitive design, their costumes, their weaving, their painting and their dancing. There were no roads into the reservation then, and I was one of the first visitors ever to see the Hopi Snake Dance. I was free to do whatever I liked. Every day I'd go to the second floor of Hopi House, where the costumes were kept, and dress to my heart's content. One day I'd be a Hopi maiden, one day I'd be the daughter of a Navajo chief. We were standing about watching a ceremonial, I in Hopi costume, when Paderewski stepped down from the Hopi House porch and gave us each a quarter. Me, too! For once, my long black hair had come in handy. The Indian girls twisted it with twine on a wooden frame, dressing it in the style they call "the squash blossom," sign of an unmarried Hopi girl. Strangely enough, where I had never found it easy to make friends, I liked the Indians and they liked me. I had one particular friend, handsome Joe Secakuku, the local Valentino. All the Indian girls and all the lady tourists were crazy about him, but he was my friend, and it was he who taught me the Indian dances.

Instead of writing letters to my mother and father, I used to make little books with illustrations and jingle rhymes. The Indian influence is very apparent in the tale of a little "Injun . . . his name was Hopi-Joe," complete with the Hopi symbols and two fighting cocks on the cover, and in one about the *Adventures of Alkali Ike*, a cowboy, inspired no doubt by the cowboy who taught me to ride a mule (but who looked so different, so country-bumpkin when he showed up in Los Angeles in his city clothes). There were also numerous parodies of adventurers, animal and human, who wanted to see the world and always ended up in trouble — probably my way of punishing them for taking the trips I wanted to take.

But one of my ambitions was realized at the Canyon. I've

always wanted to climb mountains, Anapurna, Mt. Everest, the higher the better. One summer day Byron Harvey Jr. and I decided to follow some surveyors down into the Canyon. They didn't know we were following them and we didn't follow them too long. When we came to the famous rock formation called "The Battleship," I had a great idea. No one had ever scaled "The Battleship." We would! We borrowed some rope and ladders the surveyors had left along the road and up we went, almost *straight* up. Of course getting up was one thing, getting down another. We were still up there, surveying the world, when a hue and cry went out for Byron Harvey Jr., the son and heir of Harvey House and the Santa Fe Railroad! His tutor was on the edge of the canyon in a state of consternation; a rescue party was assembled post haste. They finally lowered us down with ropes.

School was tame after that. But when I was graduated from college, my parents were living in potash country, Trona, California; I didn't want to live where everyone was making potash, so I went to Stanford to take my master's degree in French.

And what was to become of me now that I knew French and Spanish? Now that I had my Bachelor's and my Master's?

I spent a strange restless summer at Aunt Mittie's. In October, I received a phone call from one of the most famous schools on the coast, The Bishop School for Girls at La Jolla. Their French teacher had been called back to France, they needed a substitute teacher, I'd been highly recommended by the professors at Stanford. Could I come at once?

Could I! Out of the blue, I had a life's work; a career had found me, I was a schoolteacher. You could tell I was a schoolteacher: I wore a navy-blue tailored suit, starched white collars and cuffs, oxfords, and my hair tightly drawn back into a washerwoman's knot. Of course there were bangs across the front and I bought, for the trip down, a bright red racing car; but you could tell I was a schoolteacher. A woman with a career.

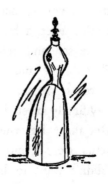

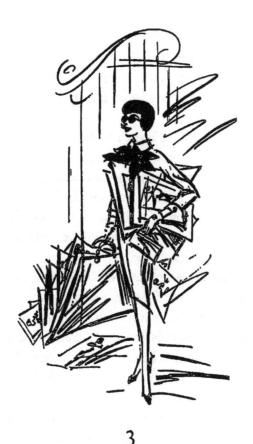

3

The Education of a Dress Doctor

THE BISHOP SCHOOL at La Jolla looks like a lovely early
California mission, quiet, cloistered, with cream-colored adobe
walls four feet thick, great Moorish arches and one imposing tower, the Bishop's. That's where I was to live, in
the Bishop's Tower! You could look out over the sea, and

every night and every morning the mellow bells sang a call to chapel. I parked my racy racing car downtown — it simply didn't have sufficient academic dignity — and walked into my new life.

My task was teaching French to thirty-five fresh-faced girls in shirtmaker uniforms with sailor collars; half of them were as old as I. I loved teaching, even that first day. The standards at Bishop were the highest, the girls the brightest, the classroom smelled somehow like all the classrooms I had known, of erasers and chalk and newly washed blackboard, of sharpened pencils and worn wood.

The morning of classes went well. The crisis came at noon. At noon I found myself heading a table of twelve French majors with whom I'd be eating all my meals and who were accustomed to speak only French at table. One of them, a girl obviously born and raised in France, turned to me and spoke rapidly in French, ending *"N'est-ce pas, Mademoiselle?"*

Mademoiselle flushed to the edge of her bangs. I'd had nine years of academic French; I could conjugate the pluperfect of any verb, read the most archaic literature, recite whole verses from the *Chanson de Roland*; my French was magnificent but my accent strictly Los Angeles — if I opened my mouth now I'd be dead. Worse: I'd be alive tomorrow, facing a classroom over which I'd lost control.

"Do you know, Suzanne," I said quickly, "I think you need practice in speaking English more than in speaking French. Wouldn't it be fairer to Suzanne, girls, if we spoke English at table?" And we did, for the rest of the semester.

If they made sacrifices for me, I made some for them, too. As a member of the faculty, I chaperoned the dances. Near as we were to San Diego, our dances were well attended by dashing young service men, and I, who longed to dance, who had indeed won a huge almost-silver loving cup, had to sit primly against the wall with the rest of the faculty and watch.

Chaperoning the girls on their Saturday excursions to San Diego was more fun. Each teacher took turns escorting the seniors into town for matinees, symphony concerts and recitals. All very cultural. One Saturday, as we wandered about waiting for symphony time, the girls suggested we "attend" the concert . . . by way of Tijuana. I'd boasted how well I could speak Spanish; why didn't I take them across the border and show them? One of the girls had a car; in nothing flat we were on our way. I shudder to think what might have happened. Suppose we'd had a flat tire on the lonely road? Been arrested? Been hit over the head and dragged into a sinister marijuana den? We weren't. We wandered about the sunlit streets, looked at all the curios, ate enchiladas and came home safe and sound.

We were never found out, either. I was able to finish the semester with honor. When the authentic French teacher returned, I cranked up my car (it had leather upholstery but no self-starter) and sailed off armed with recommendations that easily secured me another post, in Los Angeles this time: the Hollywood School for Girls.

It was a most unusual school. Every student had some

connection with the motion picture industry. My pupils included Agnes, Cecilia and Katherine de Mille. Every time de Mille was shooting a big scene at the studio, school closed down and we went over to Paramount to watch. Then someone else's father or uncle would start a picture and we'd go to join the fun. That's the kind of school it was; we gave everyone good grades and flunked no one. (As it happened, the de Mille girls were bright — they'd have passed at Bishop!) My job was teaching all grades, fifth through high school, French and — Art.

Art certainly wasn't one of my subjects; to keep one jump ahead of them, I'd read *The History of Art* every night and teach it the next day, give them problems to execute and criticize their work. Then I decided I needed to know more about art, so I went first to Otis, then to Chouinard Art School. I took everything at once — seascape, landscape, water color, mechanical drawing — showing absolutely no aptitude at anything. It didn't matter; I wasn't trying to become an artist, I was trying to keep one jump ahead of my classes.

At Chouinard one of my classmates was Betty Head, and at one of our school dances I met her brother, Charles, who'd just graduated from college and was doing research work at the Bakersfield oil fields. He was a brilliant young man with every promise of a bright future and we were married after a long, rather intellectual correspondence. It was a marriage disrupted first by separation, then by Charles's illness, and eventually by his death. In the beginning, he continued his work at Bakersfield and I continued teaching at Hollywood School for Girls.

During summer vacation that year, looking for a summer job, I answered a want ad placed by Howard Greer, head designer at Paramount, who was looking for a sketch artist. I wrote for an appointment and received an answer: I was to be at the studio the next morning at ten, bringing sketches. That night I made the rounds at Chouinard and collected the cream — all the students' best landscapes, seascapes, oils, watercolors, sketches, life, art, everything. Howard Greer looked at the sketches and said he'd never seen so much talent in one portfolio. "Report tomorrow for work," he said, "your salary will be fifty dollars a week." Fifty dollars a week looked like a fortune to a schoolteacher earning fifteen hundred dollars a year. The next day I was sitting in front of a drawing board staring at a blank piece of paper on which I was to sketch evening dresses and riding habits. I sat there a long time. I'd figured I could fake it, but . . .

"What's the matter?" Howard said.

"Don't know how to draw!"

"But all those wonderful sketches in your portfolio!" he said.

"Borrowed," I said.

Instead of firing me, Howard started teaching me to sketch. He thought the whole thing very funny.

I should mention that I thought I'd showed up at the

studio looking exactly like a sketch artist: black suit, white blouse, a huge black tie to help suggest the Latin Quarter, sheer hose, high-heeled patent pumps to suggest Hollywood. But this is the way Howard has described our meeting: "We placed an ad in the papers and a young girl with a face like a pussycat crossed with a Fujita drawing appeared with a carpetbag full of sketches." He always insisted I looked like the Japanese artist Fujita: I insisted I did not — Fujita had a mustache. One night, however, Howard gave a big masquerade party; I went as Fujita, complete with mustache, and everyone recognized me at once!

From the first day at the studio, I was fascinated, enthusiastic and willing, but I hadn't the least notion that I'd ever survive. To this moment I wonder why I did. Perhaps because I worked hard and was willing to tackle anything — paint polka dots on china silk butterfly wings for *Peter Pan*, paint shoes with printed patterns to match the printed gowns to be worn by a Gloria Swanson or a Jetta Goudal. (We all turned out when the great Gloria, then the Marquise de la Falaise de Coudray, returned to the studio after a honeymoon trip to Europe; we threw roses — given us by the studio for the purpose — as she stepped from her leopard-lined limousine.) One day when I wasn't busy, Frank Richardson, head of Wardrobe, stopped by.

"We're taking inventory," he said. "If you've nothing to do at the moment, why don't you count the beads, the button molds and the jewels?"

These were all kept in fruit jars and little boxes on the

very top shelf. There was one jar of square-inch jet, one jar of pearls, etc. I spent *days* on the stepladder counting beads. Finally Mr. Richardson came to see what had happened to me.

"Mr. Richardson," I said proudly, "see this jar? It has four hundred and ninety-three square–cut jets!"

How he laughed. He'd meant for me to count the jars and boxes, not each individual bead!

I spent time in the workroom watching patterns being made. After a fitting, I'd ask the girls why there had been changes. I'd never sewed, and it was a long way from the hemstitching mother had taught me to the intricacies of sewing which you must understand if you're ever going to design a dress that can be made.

Also, of course, I was learning to sketch. At Chouinard at night, I abandoned my fancy oil and watercolor work for humble sketching, learning to draw the human figure. I studied everything Howard Greer and Travid Banton did. They both did most of their own sketches in those days, handling one picture at a time, where today I do a quick little *croquis* — pencil sketch thumbnail size — and my sketch artist interprets them into full size drawings; but we handle five and six pictures at a time.

Luckily, I was a quick student. Within six months, I could sketch in the style of Greer or in the style of Banton so that it was impossible to tell that someone else had done it. I was one of the "little things" that sat in the back room. There were three or four "little things" at three or four easels, and we sat busy with our chores (with time out for an occasional game of jacks). When Howard designed a beaded dress for Pola Negri, he had me draw in the beads. I started to draw *each* bead until he explained . . . "Look, Edith, pretend you're a trained fly." When he saw the feathers I was drawing on the sketch of his ostrich dress for Irene Rich, he just sighed and said my feathers looked like tired spaghetti. He and Travis taught me constantly; I couldn't have stayed on a week without them. They were both very young, very amused by me and very patient. I'd never had much faith in myself and now I was completely unsure.

As I was working away on my spaghetti feathers one afternoon, the great, great Jetta Goudal wandered out of the big fitting room into the cubbyhole where we worked. I looked over my glasses at this vision in silver lamé and chinchilla. . . . It was floating toward me. . . . It stood beside me. . . . It looked over my shoulder. Silence. . . . Then a deep, thrilling voice said:

"Little sketch girl, never draw anything like that for me!" I couldn't even answer, I just went into shock.

Every moment threatened to be my last. There is no place at a studio for people who don't know what they're doing, so you can't say you don't know, or ask how. My first big assignment was to do the Candy Ball costumes for Cecil B. de Mille's *The Golden Bed*. I drew girls dressed as lollypops, peppermint sticks, chocolate drops. Howard asked me if I knew how the designs could be executed and I assured him they were simple. So he took the rather amusing sketches to Mr. de Mille, who promptly okayed them.

Then came the crisis. I'd drawn very elongated girls with bodies like peppermint sticks and fingernails of peppermint sticks two feet long. I was called out to the workroom to supervise the making. Bluffing, I called for long underwear, better yet, leotards. I spread them on the floor and painted stripes on them using a can of red paint. It didn't work. The minute the leotards were put on, the stripes wiggled and waved. I called for a professional model. On her we put a skintight leotard and painted the stripes on. Unfortunately we used red house paint, and it didn't dry. The poor girl stood for three hours waiting for those stripes to dry; then she couldn't stand any longer. We removed the leotard, the stripes ran together, the model was sent to the hospital to recover.

Now for the candy-cane fingernails two feet long. I got thimbles for all ten fingers of each girl, pulled striped silk gloves over the thimbles, punctured holes in the thimbles and inserted the peppermint sticks.

Came the day of shooting and, shortly after, came a blast from Mr. de Mille — who was never a patient man. The peppermint sticks had started cracking during the dance routines. Using real candy proved to be a mess. I'd put candy on their heads, on their shoulders; whenever they got within a half a foot of each other, the candy would stick. From that day on, I've never drawn anything I couldn't *make*.

For a long time I did tasseled headdresses for elephants, trappings for horses, monkeys, chimpanzees, poodles and camels. We did some big Biblical pictures with lots of animals. One nasty camel about to dwell on the Ark actually spit at me. No one'd told me camels spit! I found elephants very unco-operative, too. They have complexes about clothes and are inclined to pull off all trappings with their trunks. They hated me *and* my clothes, and I would gladly have swapped them for my dear old burros back in Searchlight. I've never gotten completely away from animals. I did a whole wardrobe for Joan Fontaine's poodle in *The Emperor Waltz*, and one of my most difficult patients was the cat who played "Rhubarb."

A junior designer does whatever no one else has time for. While Travis Banton and Howard Greer coped with the stars, I did some of the best-dressed animals on the screen — the idiot nieces, grandmothers, and maids, graduating slowly to the "B" westerns, the language of the divided skirt. Incidentally, it was like a course in master strategy to watch Greer and Banton handle their star clients. Howard was very serious with Pola Negri; Travis was gay and bantering with Carole Lombard; no two actresses were treated the same way, and this was the day when the studio really catered to a name. If she chose to tear up a dress, she tore it up.

Redheaded Nancy Carroll did just that. She was an important star. I was watching Travis fit her — there was no temper tantrum, no discussion. She took one look at herself in the dress and calmly *ripped* it off. Had I been the designer I'd have screamed, I'm sure. Travis calmly walked out of the room. P.S. Nancy wore that dress in the picture. I made a mental note of the whole procedure and added it to my education.

Money was nothing at the time, but Travis was maintaining his authority. And when I say money was nothing . . . this was the era B.B. (Before Budgets). A star's wardrobe for a picture included her handmade lingerie, whatever the lady wanted. Once, when Greer was in Europe and Banton on vacation, THE PRESENCE walked in, Garbo. She was carrying a beautiful man's bathrobe she wished made over to fit her. This was my privilege.

For my first "B" western, I sketched my heroine in a homespun, button-down-the-front dress, properly demure. The director insisted that the dress be low-necked. I, with a schoolmarm's precision, insisted that pioneer women hadn't worn low-necked dresses across the plains.

"Edith," he said, "you don't know the facts of life. If women hadn't worn low-necked dresses, your grandmother and mother wouldn't have been born and neither would you." I'd just lost the first of a hundred battles. My heroine not only wore a low-necked dress across the plains, she survived an Indian raid, fire, famine, flood and a broken wagon-axle without soiling her crisp white collars and cuffs. As one eminent reviewer wrote, *This* [referring to my heroine's décolletage homespun] *is what makes Hollywood ridiculous.*

"Back to schoolteaching," I thought.

But I stayed on, learning to buck what a Hollywood designer must try to buck: first the star who puts herself in your hands but knows exactly what she wants, then the producer and the director, either of whom is likely to say, "I want a square neckline, my wife always wears one," the sound man who doesn't like the rustle, the color consultant who worries himself sick about plaids and tweeds (especially today on wide-screen), the art director who insists "You can't use blue, the interior of my room is blue," the set decorator who screams, "Oh, my God, you can't use a black dress for this scene, I've planned a black sofa!" . . . or the front office reminding you, as the day of economy came in, ugliest of all words, WE CAN'T AFFORD . . . or, finally, the censor who may decree that *mousseline de soie* is too diaphanous. . . . The designer wages a losing war. To win, you'd have to be a combination of psychiatrist, artist, fashion designer, dressmaker, pincushion, historian, nursemaid and purchasing agent.

But a designer I wanted to be. For the first time, at the studio, I began to take on positive color. I had a flair for flamboyance — remember my fire-engine-red car, my dress-up as Navajo princess or Hopi heroine? — and these were the days when Hollywood was a Barnum and Bailey world. An actress was far more interested in being beautiful than in looking a part; the screen plays themselves were fantasies rather than realities; as for design, it was the era of gold bathtubs, ermine bathrobes; every working girl wore high-fashion satins dripping with mink; Anna May Wong wore her gold fingernails inches long, and exotic kimonos to match. Designers tried to outdo each other. I caught the flavor and the fever.

When Mr. de Mille wanted a "different" riding habit for Irene Rich, I sketched a beautiful side-saddle habit. Howard Greer smiled. "We can't use this," he said, "it would look just like something everyone would wear." So I took some gold paint and painted the boots, the whip and the hat into gleaming gold, and Howard and Mr. de Mille both liked it very much. I was in Never-Never Land.

There were a few heartaches, too. I dressed Pola Negri once, she was one of the top stars, I longed to do something fabulous, the script limited me to a peasant woman's black skirt and shawl.

I had a chance at Gladys Swarthout when a "B" picture scheduled for me was recast and slated for bigger things; but Miss Swarthout felt that from the point of protocol I wasn't important enough to do her clothes. This happened a number of times. There were stars who wanted Howard or Travis, and in their absence would bring in their own designers from the outside.

The first picture I ever did with a major star was *The Wolf Song*, starring Lupe Velez and Gary Cooper. It was a horse opera with a Latin flavor; and for once, instead of being stuck with the Grandma or the sheriff's wife (seen in a long shot), I dressed the star. Lupe was to be a poor girl, Gary was madly in love with her; the big scene was played in moonlight, and the script called for a simple white lace dress. So — I used the whole bolt!

I was trying to impress Miss Velez, the first star I'd ever really met, who was unhappy to begin with because she'd expected Howard Greer to do her clothes. The fact that I spoke fluent Spanish helped me. So did the white lace dress.

Lupe loved it. Instead of looking like a simple country girl, she looked as if she were about to be presented at the Court of Isabella. This couldn't happen today — but in those days, we didn't screen-test clothes and no one saw this concoction except Lupe and me until it was time to shoot the scene. It certainly surprised the director! It took a huge truck to transport that dress to location, and Lupe could barely move once she was in it. In those days, nobody minded except one intelligent critic, who wrote: *If there hadn't been so much dress, there would have been more scene.*

I seriously considered going back to teaching. The only reason I didn't, I guess, was that I was beginning to discover what to me is magic — that you can actually change a person with clothes. (Inadvertently, I'd just made Lupe Velez look sophisticated and worldly, where she should have looked demure and puritan.) To convey character by dress was something with which to experiment; and, like any young intern in his first hospital, I became fascinated with my experiments. I never dreamed that over the years I'd be able to use as guinea pigs the most beautiful women in the world.

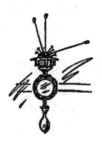

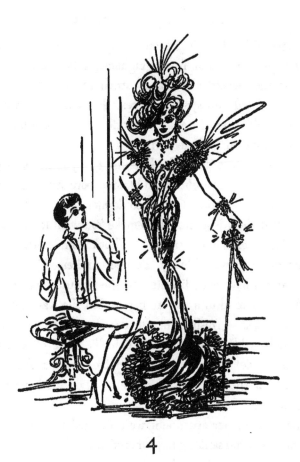

4

Patients Who Taught Me

I WENT UP to see her sometime — up to her apartment, as
a matter of fact — to take her measurements and plan the costumes for *She Done Him Wrong.* Howard Greer had left
Paramount to open his own salon; Travis Banton was in
Europe on business; I was completely on my own for the

first time with a big picture and a big, big star: Mae West. It was quite a switch from ginghams, calicos and divided skirts to the velvets, satins and ostrich feathers which Miss West translated into symbols of sex. I might say it was this schoolmarm's advent into a new world where every little texture had a meaning all its own.

I learned to be a doctor by listening to my patients — Mae West, for example, taught me all I know about sex, clotheswise. "I love fabric I can feel, Honey; so do men." . . . "They like clothes that show just enough to make 'em want to see more." . . . "Low necklines stylish? They're imperative!" . . . "Without diamonds, Honey, I'd feel undressed," she said. She may not have been literate, but she was utterly articulate; she'd never starred in a picture before, but she was absolutely sure of herself — fresh from the Broadway hit of *Diamond Lil*, which she'd written and of which *She Done Him Wrong* was the movie version. She looked like no one else; she'd have died if she had! She'd *created* a style for herself and stuck with it.

The floors of her apartment were covered with polar bear rugs in which you sank up to your ankles, the draperies were of heavy white satin, the walls mirrored, the lamps were white porcelain statues of Mae, and the most imposing "statue" in the place was La West herself, in white satin negligee with a train four yards long. She dropped the negligee, and the girls measured: 38-24-38, a full-bodied woman with perfect alabaster skin, magnificent bosom, shoulders and arms which she believed in baring at all times. Her theory: "If it's worth seeing, show it." She wore no bra, no corsets; we'd have no figure problems; for the period costumes, we'd need only to bone the bodice of each dress.

"I like 'em tight, girls," she said; and tight they were, there wasn't a costume in which she could lie, bend or sit, and I was sure that she could *breathe* only when I saw her survive the picture. To afford her some small relaxation, we improvised a reclining board; it had armrests and was tilted at an angle, and there she'd lean between scenes in glittering splendor, the jewels winking from her hourglass gowns and dazzling from her throat, ears, wrists, and every finger.

I designed thirty or forty pounds of jewelry for Mae to wear as "Diamond Lil." I first found pictures of period jewelry to show her. "Fine, Honey," she said, "just make the stones *bigger*." The period of the picture was one of the most beautiful in the world fashionwise, and she was the one woman of the modern world who could offer the figure needed to round those fashions out. There was a walking costume of lace and ostrich feathers with a lace parasol to match. ("It may not keep the sun off, but it's awful pretty.") There was a white costume of satin embroidered in diamonds and trimmed with ostrich feathers and a dust ruffle of tulle. Her very favorite was a jeweled black satin worn with an ostrich feather boa. I spent half my time at Cawston's Ostrich Farm in South Pasadena ordering ostrich feathers, riding in carts that were trundled about the place by trained ostriches.

She loved satin, velvet, silk that felt glamorous — never wool; and she was very responsive to color — black, white, purples, violets. Green? Never! Pearls? Never! Pearls, she said, meant sorrow; green, she said, meant bad luck. We replaced the green taffeta I'd inadvertently made with a black satin hung in jet. (When Shirley Booth came along years later, she also had a prejudice about green. She had worn a green dress in her first stage success; green to her means good luck!)

For one scene, Mae said: "I don't have much to say here, Edith, let's do something with this dress so at least they won't notice what anyone else is saying." So we designed six swallows, big as cups, and outlined in brilliants, to fly from the left-hand waistline to the right shoulder. No one did notice what anyone else said in that scene!

For another sequence, we needed a vampirish negligee. I made a skin-tight black nightgown and over it a chiffon-and-diamond negligee that gave the effect of a spider web. On the shoulder I perched a huge diamond spider, anchored on with adhesive tape. When Mae wore this onto the set, the whistles and screams sounded as if the *Queen Mary* were docking in New York Harbor. Mae had switched the diamond spider — to a more strategic spot. It took a half-hour to quiet the hilarity and get Cary Grant, Gilbert Roland and the crew back to work.

This picture started a whole new mode in Paris. *La Vogue Mae West*, they called it, with feathers on hats, feather boas, velvet and satin gowns, the hourglass, totally lush, seductive look. And I, as a young intern, was even more influenced than the Paris mode. Mae West had taught me what a woman can do with a format.

She was superbly herself; fashion could go hang. Nor was there ever an apology, no "It's too bad I'm so short," or "If only I were thinner!" Behind the silken slink was the iron structure of a bright businesswoman and a bright businesswoman's fine mind. She knew what she knew, and made the most of it: the highest of high heels, the longest of skirts, the tightest of waists, bare bosom day or night, hot or cold.

On screen or off, she glorified this creature she had made of herself, keeping her humor broad but not grotesque, her style ditto. Hers was a wary sense of doing the right thing at the right time; she was never late for an appointment, she never changed one; she was informal and gay, and we became friends. Still are.

As a matter of fact, as this is being written, I am working with Mae again, for the first time in years, designing a raft of peignoirs, negligees, hostess gowns and glittery evening gowns which are totally interchangeable: she can wear them in her personal life, she can wear them, just as well, in her public appearances. Mae West is still utterly Mae West; the successful format that impressed the intern now confronts the doctor — confronts and confounds the world, for that matter. On the 1958 Academy Awards broadcast, boasting the cream of show business talent, who stole the show and the one million viewers?

Rugged individualism paid off for Mae; it paid off, too, for Clara Bow, the patient who resisted every effort of the schoolteacher to make her authentic — who gave me pointers, instead, on Flaming Youth. In an era when everyone in

America wore a straight-line dress with the "waistline" somewhere between hips and knees, Clara wore a good tight belt
at her natural waist (no matter what was designed for her),
became a star in spite of it (her fans wrote her some twenty
thousand letters a week), and spent all her spare time trying
to reform me (I've always kept an old photograph of Clara,
inscribed to me "With love, but why don't you put your g——
d—— belt around your waist where it belongs?").

Design high-fashion clothes for her, she added a belt.
Even her bathing suit had an added belt, and with it she wore
white satin pumps. When she played the part of a famous
tennis player, she wore shorts, a cute sweater, high heels.
"They make my legs look prettier," she said. In a picture where
she was portraying a young thing with no money, she insisted
on huge chandelier earrings. The director warned me, whatever I did, not to let Clara wear those earrings.

"Really, doesn't he want me to wear my earrings?" Clara
said, looking at me with that pouted underlip.

"Really," I said.

So she only wore *one* earring.

In a picture where she played a manicurist, her uniform
was of gray satin with gray satin pumps to match, and Clara
added a diamond anklet!

She wanted to look young, sexy, the symbol of Flaming
Youth. And she did, in spite of me. Actually, Clara should
have had an older designer. We were of an age and good
friends. The only way I ever won a point was to laugh
her out of her eccentricities rather than forbid them. The

eccentricities didn't matter, anyhow — Hollywood had the reputation, then, for being bizarre. What would be bad taste today was amusing at a time when you could go shopping on Hollywood Boulevard with a leopard on a leash, especially if your Rolls-Royce was upholstered in leopardskin.

What Clara was selling on the screen, she essentially was — a glamorous flapper; and what made her glamorous were her high spirits, her gaiety, her endless vitality (she wore colors to match, hot colors: flame red, pinks, burnt orange). She loved parties and gave them, inviting a weird mixture of stars, directors, college students, diplomats, politicians (once there was a prime minister), everybody. She didn't care what you did or who you were, if you were fun. She always had the furniture moved out of her house and put in the garage so there'd be room for dancing; she always hired an orchestra; and often, there'd be a motif, a Turkish party, for example, where she served shishkabob.

Her house was what you might call "early Hollywood," very elegant. One night she invited the whole USC football team. She and I planned the party together and it was a darb, as long as it lasted. I wore a fringed dress and she wore pink beaded chiffon, we danced the Charleston and had a fine time — until the football team went home. We'd forgotten that they were in training, that they had to get in early.

Oh, well, she'd just give another party! Clara took life as it came, day by day having fun, never thinking of the future. There was nothing small about her, nothing petty. In one picture, I had to dress her as a poor working girl (with a heart of gold) and dress Jean Harlow, who was playing second lead, as the rich girl (heart of stone). For their big scene together, Jean wore white satin, a white satin cape edged in sable, and around her throat ropes of pearl. She looked very beautiful and everyone said so. I was worried. Jean looked *so* very beautiful, and Clara was the star. But Clara couldn't have cared less. She thought Jean looked gorgeous and didn't mind her looking gorgeous.

They were very different girls, both very sexy. Jean the introvert, Clara the extrovert; Jean cool, Clara ebullient. Her fittings were a virtual romp, Clara holding court, her three Great Danes lounging about her feet, tripping up the fitters every time they moved.

"Hey! This makes me look like a crystal chandelier!" she'd cry, shimmying to shake the crystal drops of a beaded sheath. We compromised. She wore the "crystal chandelier" and I added ermine tails all around the bottom of her already elaborate ermine cape.

I did several pictures with Clara — she didn't object to having the assistant — she didn't care who did her clothes so long as she got what she wanted.

If Clara taught me about unreality, Charles Laughton introduced me to reality and the importance of research. The picture was *White Woman* and Mr. Laughton played a planter, whose one vanity was embroidery on his vests. The vests had to be rakish but dignified, had to set him apart from other planters. He explained with relish the psychological

implications these vests must achieve, my first living proof
that great actors feel costumes *are* essential to their portrayal!
It was unexpected news and a happy break between my usual
Western heroines and the army of bit players.

When it wasn't grandmas or maids, it was the children,
hundreds of them. It seemed to me we never did a picture
that didn't have a child for me to dress. The theatrical small
fry of Hollywood invariably wore organdy dresses three inches
above the crotch with lots and lots of ruffles, white Russian
boots, and blond curls; *and* invariably, they knew exactly how
I should dress them. So did their mamas.

One picture called for several small girls to play proper,
well-brought-up children of millionaires. The little girls were
to be impeccably dressed, the quintessence of elegance and
good taste. I dressed them in white French batiste with hand
tucks, and they did look charming. The director, a fanatic on
realism, was very much pleased, but he asked one thing more:

"Please," he said, "have the children wear the dresses home,
then have them laundered so they won't look as if they'd just
come directly from the fitting room."

The children wore the dresses home. Next morning, when
they returned, one dress was covered with lace ruffles.

"The dress looked so *poor*," the mama explained. "I guess
you didn't realize this child is supposed to be rich!"

Now, I love children; I even love mamas when they're not
in motion pictures. Once in the business, the mothers must
have explained to the little darlings that, when they come up

to see Miss Head, they should be as nice as possible, smile as sweetly as possible, then Miss Head would make them a pretty dress. They evidently figured that the wider they smiled, the prettier the dress, because every child arrived showing her teeth, jaws clenched.

With one exception. . . . A very small girl came in one day before making her screen debut in *Little Miss Marker;* she had quite a few changes of costume, and one transformed her into a little medieval princess. For the first time I had a youngster in my fitting room who was not a moppet, who *was* a little girl; she enchanted me, as she did everyone else on the lot. Her name was Shirley Temple and it never occurred to me that she'd be a star who'd outshine Garbo and Janet Gaynor. Why, neither she nor her mother ever told me *how!*

Between the little girls who did, and the perpetual westerns, and the ermine tails on Clara's wrap, and the petals on top of endless petals, I sometimes felt as dizzy as an intern at his first operation. More than once I was about to give notice.

The patient who really influenced me to stay was Carole Lombard. Here was an exciting girl with a flair for fashion, a casual elegance, the ability to stimulate fashion — what she wore on the screen, women copied. I was familiar enough with the exotics, the Negris, the Swansons, the Wests, the Bows; here was something quite different: the first fashion-conscious star I'd met, one who could influence the taste of the American woman.

Carole loved tailored clothes; she hated dresses that looked, she said, "like a cross between French pastry and a lampshade." This was for me. I took a deep breath and designed my first suits for Carole to wear, in a picture where she played a smart super-secretary. I also had to do one "lampshade" dress of tulle (which she couldn't abide), but for a purpose — the dress had to be fluffy and floaty and then get limp in the rain.

"I know you don't like this type of dress," I said, hesitantly, "what should we do?"

Carole laughed. "I don't like hoopskirts, either, but if we were doing *Birth of a Nation* I guess I'd have to wear the damned things."

At least, that's *sort* of what she said. She actually used the most colorful language of any human I've ever met, with a purpose, I'm sure. It was part of her individualism.

She couldn't have found a quicker common denominator. The girls in the workroom worshiped her, the fitters begged to work with her. That's a true barometer. Back in the workroom, when you announce a star is coming in, there'll sometimes be a groan and a moan and a "Do I have to fit HER?" . . . "Heaven help us!". . . "Let's stay home tomorrow, girls." But for Lombard they were ready, willing and able. "Let me go too, I can carry your pincushion." Her fittings were gay, hilarious, you could hear them six blocks off. She had great clothes sense and a true clotheshorse figure, but she didn't take clothes or herself seriously. Nothing was sacred, not even the third act of *Camille;* nothing was a crisis.

With her, I realized for the first time how important a designer is, not only to an actress, but to women. Anyone can do a pioneer character woman and make her look old, worn and travel-weary; anyone can do a trapeze artist or a clown; but to actually work in the medium of contemporary clothes and help with the development of a personality — that, to me, was exciting. I'd seen Travis Banton, in the years he'd worked with Carole, transform her from a salesgirl to a duchess, all in modern dress. Now, in his absence, I was doing it, creating little sheath suits that enhanced her lean, clean greyhound look. I've loved suits ever since, *and* the Lombard look. I began to realize what you could do with smart clothes. Like any novice I began to dream of miracles.

I was single-handed going to someday turn Hollywood into a vision of superbly, immaculately dressed women like Carole Lombard. What a woman wears, I felt, sets the pace for what she says and does. In a print dress at a luncheon, she'd be different than in svelte décolletage sipping champagne. What she wears conveys who she is. Carole in a Clara Bow dress would be one thing, in a Mae West dress, something else, in one of her own chic, sheathlike suits — Carole Lombard.

There was a magic power in clothes. They could develop peronality. I decided to stick with them.

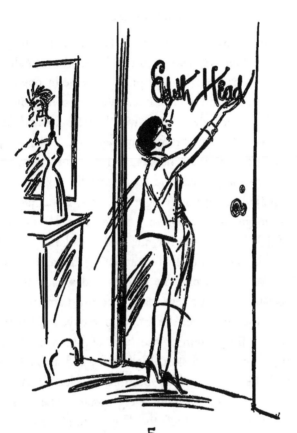

5
The Doctor Hangs up Her Shingle

FIRST OF THE jungle pictures so dear to an era of escapism
was *The Jungle Princess* (1936). For it I designed a garment
that was to become a national institution — the "sarong." Not
the *authentic* sarong, you understand, an authentic sarong,
wrapped below the waistline, wouldn't clear any censor! My

unauthentic version was made of bright, mad red, printed with white hibiscus; and to fill it Paramount conducted a nationwide search for a jungle princess. One by one the state finalists were sent up to my clinic. We'd dress each one in the same sarong, tuck the same white blossom behind her ear and slip the same shell bracelets on her arm. Then the pretty native would go over for her screen test. They were all very pretty, very voluptuous, and to me totally uninteresting. I wasn't prejudiced against jungle aspirants, I was just not interested in jungle sarongs any more than I was in westerns. High fashion was for me; and I had no idea, at the moment, that I'd eventually be translating the sarong into high fashion evening gowns, play clothes and what have you — all associated with the legendary Dorothy Lamour.

Among the candidates she arrived one day, a girl with dark hair twisted into a bun at the back of her head. She was wearing a sweater and skirt, high heels, and a shoulder-strap bag, and she was incredibly beautiful — clear, creamy magnolia skin, big blue eyes and a big bosom. The minute she took off her sweater, half the "big bosom" came with it! Falsies! She kicked off her shoes, pulled down her luxuriant hair and the red sarong was wrapped around her.

Now a sarong has neither hooks nor eyes, it stays up on certain natives simply because they are well endowed by nature to hold it up. Dorothy was younger than she admitted at the time, and she was *not* well enough endowed. We helped fill the sarong out to the proper proportions and used adhesive tape to hold it in place. Dorothy was completely enthusiastic about the effect. So were the boys on the set. Indeed, the wolf whistle originated for Dorothy Lamour the day she walked on the set to test for *Jungle Princess*. Later the boys developed a vocabulary: there were 3-whistle, 5-whistle and 20-whistle dresses; and once, when I was trying to "sell" Dottie a dress she didn't like — a high-necked, long-sleeved, covered-up white jersey for *My Favorite Brunette* — I bribed the electricians to be sure of at least a 5-whistle salute.

Because, of course, Dorothy won the contest and the role. Least voluptuous of the contestants, she became the very promise of voluptuousness and in time her figure lived up to that promise. *The Jungle Princess* made her a star overnight, and started the vogue for jungle and adventure pictures that lasted more than ten years. Long before that, Dottie was able to hold up her own sarong without any visible means of support!

The plots of these pictures were usually the same. She was always being chased by lions, tigers or elephants; she was fraternizing with cheetahs, crocodiles and other livestock, she was being tossed into volcanoes or facing equally volcanic adventures with Bing Crosby and Bob Hope. She made spy pictures, Road pictures (to Morocco, Singapore, Utopia, Zanzibar, Bali and Rio), and other pictures where she symbolized the alluring adventuress. Luckily, she was afraid of nothing and took it all in stride, the animals, the waterfalls and the hilarious leading men. Thrown off cliffs and eaten by tigers, she emerged unscathed except for an unfortunate case of mange she caught from the tiger Satan. And she added a happy zest to life on the Paramount lot.

Everyone loved Dottie because she had no delusions of

being Sarah Bernhardt. She was strictly Dorothy Lamour, ex-girl singer with Herbie Kaye's band, ex-elevator operator, and perfectly content to be doing just what she was doing. She would stand poised on the brink of a volcano, fling herself to the "gods" to save her "people," and five minutes later be back in her dressing room safe and sound, munching chocolate and playing gin rummy.

From the moment her first picture was released, we were deluged with mail from tropical islands explaining that Polynesians do not wrap their sarongs above their waists, that real sarongs are made of tapa cloth; but Dorothy in her silk sarong became the household Polynesian. During the war, when silks were scarce, her sarongs were remade over and over.

Dorothy became one of the biggest names in pictures, but I never realized that until I went to Washington with her during the war. Our train was met by a motorcycle escort, there were vice presidents, senators and foreign dignitaries in the cheering section; the Army and Navy turned out . . . for Dorothy Lamour, the gay jolly girl who wanted a husband and family much more than she wanted stardom! I remember when she and Bill Howard were first married and living on the base at San Bernardino where he was stationed. They had no kitchen; Dorothy was learning to cook. I'd go down to the base with scissors, sarongs and sketches, food Dorothy wanted from the Farmer's Market and all my best recipes. We'd cook on a hot plate and wash dishes in the bathtub.

I did all of Dorothy's clothes, her screen clothes, her personal wardrobe, the wedding gown of pale blue with its slight sarong drape, the suits she wore on the war bond drives (with draped turbans), the occasional high-fashion-clothes picture like *Masquerade in Mexico*, in which Dottie got her chance at white lace and shoulder-length black gloves in the return to elegance after the war.

"This is more like it!" she cried, turning before the mirrors. "I'd begun to think I was going to have to make a career out of that jungle kimono!"

She'd spoken too soon. She did make a career of it. And I, today, am probably the most conservative designer in Hollywood because I lived through pictures like *The Road to Morocco* and Dorothy's pride-of-the-harem clothes. She and I were growing up together in the early days; we never had time to catch our respective breaths, since she made never less than four or five pictures a year.

In the middle of Dottie Lamour's second hectic year, I became head designer at Paramount: the first woman designer in the business, the first designer with a mining-camp instead of a European background. The studio sent me to Paris to complete my education, to sop up the essence of the great *couturiers* and come back ready for all contingencies; the fact that I was to be a woman designing for women, who usually prefer men, was not the least of those contingencies. Howard Greer and Travis Banton had written pages and pages of advice — WHAT TO DO IN PARIS — and luckily I had a chance to travel with Lillian Farley, a noted model who had married Frank Farley, head of the Paramount office in Paris, where Lillian was now working for *Harper's Bazaar*.

With Lillian as guide and mentor, I was able to enter every

salon as something more than a tourist, and certainly *not* as
Paramount's designer. So far as I knew, they'd never heard
of Paramount, or Hollywood. In our brief moments in New
York I'd already discovered that, fashionwise, Hollywood was
regarded as something less than barbarian.

In Paris, we visited every collection, sometimes two a day.
In between times, I looked at fabrics. I was fascinated, awed
and overcome by this first plunge into the world of fashion.
I met such designers as Alix, Schiaparelli and Balenciaga;
Lillian knew them well. I absorbed them and their creations
as I'd absorbed languages at Stanford — relentlessly. Once
or twice I murmured something about the *Folies-Bergère* and
Maxim's, but Lillian only said, "That you can do later." *That*
I never did at all; there wasn't time.

Lillian also said that it would be nice if I bought something,
people usually did. So I bought something at every house.
Carmel Snow, the famous editor of *Harper's Bazaar*, was often
at the same collections. She was very chic with her white
hair; she was, also, about my size, so anything she ordered,
I ordered, plus anything else that was "the prettiest."

I knew nothing about the facts of life or customs — the difference in tax between a plain dress or an embroidered dress,
the varied tariffs for silks, wools, cottons, etc. I just stuffed
all my lovely expensive clothes into a huge wardrobe trunk
and sailed for home. At the dock in New York, I stood under
the big H and waited for the Customs official. If I had expected him to be as impressed with my purchases as I was,
I erred. He was much *more* impressed, so impressed I had

to call the Paramount offices in New York to come bail me out. I owed hundreds and hundreds of dollars in taxes! When the Customs man found the thirty or forty lapel watches I was bringing to the girls on our staff, he wanted to know was I wholesaler or retailer?

But the Parisian excursion was not in vain. My first picture as head designer was *Café Society* with Madeleine Carroll. Here I tangled for the first time with a member of the international set, an English beauty who had, until then, been dressed by the greatest designers in Europe, and was completely at home with *haute couture.* The snobbery of fashion is a potent weapon and I blessed every moment I'd spent in the Paris salons. When she tossed *"robe de style"* or *"gilet,"* I could handle it! A good designer doesn't copy other designers; you use *couturiers,* rather, as you would a good cook book's glossary of terms — each stands for a type of dress: the draped, the bouffant, the fluid line. I was able to tab, at a glance, Madeleine Carroll's hat (Daché), her jewels (Cartier), her suit (Molyneux). It all helped.

I mapped out my strategy like a general. Nothing was accidental. The Clinic was remodeled in gray like the French salons. I adopted a simple, unobtrusive uniform — tailor-made suits for the most part, in monotone colors — I don't want patients looking at my figure, I want to look at theirs; when they gaze into the mirrors at a glamour production, I should be the background. I worked out my clinical approach. Doctor and patient both read the script. The story is your

Bible; first and above all, what kind of character are we dressing?

"Miss Carroll," I would say, "how do you see this woman?" It proved to be a good approach. When I don't agree with an actress, I often compromise. I'll say No, she can't have a red satin dress with a V neckline, but she can have the V neckline and "let's make it of black wool." I never say, "You'll wear a square neckline and like it."

The skill of a doctor grows with the number of patients treated and the variety of diseases. At this point, I was a just graduated medical student, and I thanked my stars for the expert crew behind me. A designer without a good fitter might as well abandon design, stuffed models are not the same as live bodies. I had four expert fitters, and drapers, beaders, finishers, cutters, each with a staff under her. I had inherited all the best from Travis, who'd inherited most of them from Howard. I was lucky. Hell is paved with good designers who've tried to build their staff in a day.

With this staff to back me, I sailed into this high-fashion dress picture with enthusiasm and, surprisingly enough, no apprehension!

Madeleine was one of the leading actresses in Europe at this time; she had done the famous *Thirty-nine Steps;* this was her first American picture. A ravishing woman, she was without tensions, without any sense of hurry or pressure, indigenous to show business, as a rule, who never allowed herself to be upset or concerned about small things. She saved her ammunition for the big crises, and, because she was so composed, so certain everything was going to be wonderful, there was seldom a crisis. Perhaps this was possible for Madeleine because her life did not revolve around show business.

A dress picture with no story handicaps, and a beauty with no emotional handicaps — I haven't had so much fun before or since! It was the period of the *robe de style* — big, bouffant, off-the-shoulder evening gowns, utterly feminine and princess-looking.

Madeleine would look at herself in the mirrors and say, "Oh, how lovely, let's have a party," and we'd have a party. She was crazy about food, authoritative about it. She introduced us to an Italian drink, Fernet Branca, guaranteed to save you on the day you want to kill yourself. She, I'm sure, will never need to touch it. She never flutters, never comes apart, as she proved years later when we were doing *The Virginian*.

Madeleine was in England then, having first fitted all the clothes here, when suddenly Technicolor came in and *The Virginian* was switched to color. This meant all new clothes — the more extreme lines and ornamentation used in black and white would seem overdone and fussy in color. A red sheath which might be magnificent for a scene in color would have looked like a gray sack in black and white.

And it was due to start shooting within days! Madeleine flew to New York, to the Ritz. I flew to New York, to the Ritz, with cartons of clothes, trunks of clothes, and sent out an emergency call for racks on which to hang the huge skirts. The Ritz Hotel had never heard of racks, but they got them somewhere, and we turned the little ivory-and-gold suite into a dressmaking establishment. We borrowed Madeleine's favorite fitter from Hattie Carnegie, and within three days did all the clothes. Madeleine had taken it for granted that everything would work out — so, of course, it did. The bridal gown was merchandised and pictured in *Vogue*, my first recognition in a fashion magazine.

But all was not high fashion or smooth sailing. Many of the most attractive actresses came at a time and for pictures which demanded fussy clothes. Mary Martin, for example. If there is anyone slim, sleek and "Mainbocher," it is Mary Martin, but I had her for a couple of the frilliest pictures ever filmed: *The Great Victor Herbert* and *Kiss the Boys Goodbye*, in which she was all but smothered in tulle, pantalets, ruffles and curls. She loathed these pictures as much as I did; but she was fresh from her Broadway triumph in *Leave It to Me*, she'd panicked the public singing "My Heart Belongs to Daddy," so she was tabbed as a cutie-pie, and a more unhappy cutie pie you've never seen. She was in a constant state of battle with the studio, pleading for a different kind of picture, roles that would give her a chance to express her personality; but the studio was making millions and saw no reason to clip her curls.

In desperation, Mary clipped everyone else's. I didn't *have* curls but I did have a lot of hair, and at every fitting, Mary'd whip out scissors and start on my mane. She cut with abandon, but not much system, and the bob which I'd worn at half-mast soon became practically a butch haircut. My bangs were in mortal jeopardy when I started hiding the scissors. Once I got the scissors away from Mary, I let my hair grow and have never been to a barber since.

When she wasn't clipping my hair, I found her a fascinating person with a quick wit and expressive speech. She invented, to describe a clothes style, my favorite expression: *plain vanilla*. She was being given whipped-cream clothes for hot-fudge pictures, when all she wanted was plain vanilla. She knew that what she was doing was completely wrong for her, so she left the studio and went back to the theater, and to the smart clothes she loved.

The other girl who came bouncing in with curls and ruffles was Betty Hutton; but *she* was happy that way. Until she came to the studio, she'd been playing in real life, on stage and in nightclubs, the enthusiastic, volatile youngster who affects pinafores and big organdy sleeves and bows and such. Everything bounced; those were the kind of parts she played. Then, when she was finally put into more sophisticated roles, in *Stork Club*, for instance, she absorbed fashion with a mind as receptive as blotting paper.

I've never seen a more complete change in format, the more interesting because her personality remains unchanged. Betty is a restless, mercurial person who is always either very up or very down. There were times when she acted as if she were about to play *Hamlet*, there were times she was exacting — she wanted everything right, and right now — there were fittings where she was restless and hated to stand still, regardless of hems that needed taking up or sleeves that needed setting in; there were other times when she was gay and high-spirited and her fittings became a circus. She always used to bring along people, friends, friends, friends, as many as twelve. She loved an audience and played up to one. As a rule I resent anybody at a fitting; but Betty fits better with an audience; she gets into the act, the friends get into the act. There were phone messages, wires, flowers arriving constantly, more phone messages — Betty's life just followed her around. And I didn't resent it; I was fascinated observing her change from bouncy ingenue to stylish woman. She adopted white gloves, suits, the well-groomed look. She'd had no idea she had an excellent fashion figure; she got one look at herself and became so style-conscious that I doubt if she remembers ever having worn a ruffle.

Another experiment in what clothes can do — Veronica Lake. Veronica was a girl who actually wore tweeds, flat heels, bulky sweaters, her hair pulled back into a hairnet. And this was the girl we transformed with hair-do (long, blonde, falling over one eye) and clothes (long, floaty, unearthly chiffons) into a glamorous nymph, half witch. Veronica got a kick out of the transformation. "Pardon me while I put on my other head," she'd say. We'd created a personality that didn't exist, and from the moment the public saw her in *This Gun for Hire* and *I Married a Witch* they accepted that personality. It was an experiment that proved what clothes can do. Once Veronica was through work, changed into her own clothes and went out into the world, no one recognized her, ever.

Ginger Rogers, on the other hand, is such a definite personality that, although she can convincingly assume the role of child or of sophisticate, the strong personality is always Ginger. No matter how you dress her, the clothes get the stamp of her individuality. She doesn't really put on a costume as an actress would, but as a girl getting ready for a high school prom, wanting her dress to be prettiest. It's a game of make believe and, because it is, she dearly loved the first picture we did together, *The Major and the Minor*. It gave her a chance to dress up as a little girl, to be funny.

The big moment in the picture was the one in which Ginger had to change from a young woman to a child, and she had to do it *on camera*. To show how the transformation could work, I dressed a little eighteen-inch mannequin and gave an exhibition for Ginger, the director and the producer. I designed a traveling suit with straight lines, a rather longish pleated skirt and a smart belted jacket with lapels that opened clear to the waistline, showing a deep V of blouse; in the neck of the blouse, a polka-dot ascot. Ginger would wear a simple broad-brimmed hat, slightly drooping, with tailored gray bow in front; plain pumps, medium-heeled.

On camera, we started the transition at the top. Ginger took her hat, flipped up the brim, ripped the bow, let the ribbon hang down in streamers. She fastened the silk shirt up at the neck and made the ascot into a big pussy-cat bow under her chin. The belted jacket was unbelted and buttoned up to the pussy-cat bow. She tucked her skirt in until it came just below the knees, using the jacket belt around the waist to pull it up. And the Major thought she *was* a Minor!

Little wonder, really. Ginger never *will* grow old, she has some element of clear spring in her chemistry. With one of the best figures in Hollywood, she can and does wear the beaded ball gown, but she loves the gingham dress.

Now when an actress says, "Come on over to my house between five and eight tonight, some friends are dropping by . . . ," you automatically assume it's a tea party or a cocktail party, depending on her state of health. Ginger lives right above me, off Coldwater Canyon; she could throw rocks into my back yard; but this was an invitation, and I dressed. "When in doubt," I always say, "a little black dress." I wore it: a black cocktail dress, white hat, white gloves. And Ginger screamed when she opened the door. She'd forgotten to say this was an *ice cream party!*

"You aren't going to mix sodas in that!" she screamed. I took a quick look at the busy soda fountain, at my hostess in her gingham dress, open-shirted men in sandals and bare-legged women in dirndls, and promptly removed hat and gloves.

Ginger is like her party — apple-pie American. When she took the Gertrude Lawrence role in *Lady in the Dark,* she did not imitate Gertrude Lawrence. She was strictly her own American self, Ginger Rogers, but this time in terms of a sophisticated woman in high-fashion clothes. For the number "Jenny Made Her Mind Up," where she imagined herself like something in a circus, behind bars of a cage, we made a mink skirt, split up the front and solidly lined in ruby glitter.

Her famous legs were encased in long sheer tights. Under a mink jacket was a blaze of the same ruby glitter. It was one of the most lavish dresses ever made in Hollywood: the mink alone cost fifteen thousand dollars; and I still show it at fashion shows as a sample of the luxury that existed before the era of budgets and economy.

Only certain shades of mink photograph correctly, and at one point the floor of my entire suite was covered with hundreds of minkskins. Director Mitch Leisen, Ginger and I studied the minks and picked out the most photogenic, Ginger sitting among them, stroking them like a child. But, mink dress or gingham, my clothes never changed Ginger's personality, she changed *them*. She even made me *eat* the fancy-colored soda I concocted at her house that day.

Talk about taking your own medicine!

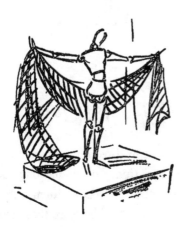

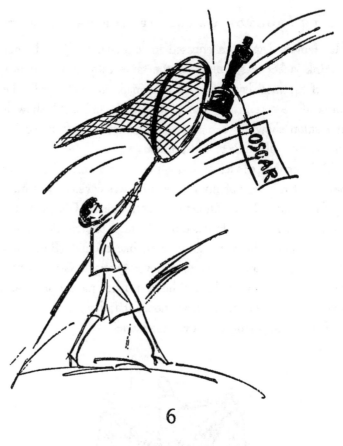

6

The First Oscar

SOME ACTRESSES fit in three minutes, some take three days. The subjective actress thinks of clothes only as they apply to her; the objective actress thinks of them only as they affect others, as a tool for the job. There are those who stand before the mirror absorbing each minute adjustment. Barbara Stanwyck is the one who stood with her back to the mirror! As for fashion, she couldn't have cared less. Up to the time we met, she had appeared in underworld pictures, show-business pictures, or intense dramas in which she could wear the sports clothes she loved: riding clothes, sweaters and skirts, shirts open at the throat, the man-tailored suit, medium heels. High fashion had never occurred to her, personally or professionally.

"I wear mostly full skirts and sweaters. I don't like hats. I hate brown," said this new patient at our first conference.

I listened as you do to symptoms. *The Lady Eve* was strictly a *dress* picture, and I was about to inoculate her with flattering furs, evening sheaths and diamonds!

Barbara walked about while director Preston Sturges explained her dual role as two sophisticated ladies: a titled Englishwoman, a lady gambler. Any diagnostic eye could tell there'd be no difficulty in Stanwyck's carrying high fashion. She's small, but she has excellent carriage, a good figure, an innate poise. She listened to our diagnosis and said nothing. Barbara would make a first-rate hand at poker.

Her first fitting involved an evening gown for the love scene with Henry Fonda. It was of clinging black crepe, a sheath with the slimmest of slim looks (she *hated* tight skirts), the lowest of necklines, a very high, very tight cummerbund (she *hates* anything tight around her midriff), and a short jacket covered with black glitter.

When she finally turned around toward the mirror and *saw* herself side view first — "More people look at you sideways or walking away, how many people see you straight on?" —

she was stunned. And she fell in love with high fashion! I worked on all Stanwyck's pictures for years. *The Lady Eve*, with its twenty-five sophisticated costumes, not only altered the type of picture Barbara did but, eventually, the way she dressed in private life as well. For a brief while she kept to her casual, tailored look personally. Then one night, as she tells it . . .

"I went with Taylor to the première of his new picture. The girl fans broke down the barricades and mobbed Bob. I was still clutching his arm when a policeman yanked me away.

" 'Okay, young lady, let the man have room to breathe!'

"When we tried to explain who I was, the officer just shook his head.

" 'Don't look like a movie star to me!'

"I went right home and phoned Edith . . .'"

It was the beginning of a long and happy relationship. I enjoyed it, because Barbara, with her clean-cut, arresting beauty, wears clothes well; but she has a sense of humor that keeps her from ever taking fashion too seriously. She's extraordinarily honest: "This looks pretty repulsive on me, don't you agree?" . . . Brutally frank: "It may be winter-white jersey, Edith; it looks like long underwear to me." . . . There is no equivocation or beating around the bush; she doesn't say "Oh, yes" to you and then tell the director, "I wouldn't be caught dead in *that!*" . . . And she's absolutely loyal. If she feels something is right, no one can change her mind. She'll stand up against director, producer and writer, come hell or high pressure.

In *Great Man's Lady* she played the owner of a gambling hall, one of the richest women in the early West. I copied a dress worn by a noted woman of the period: black velvet embroidered with diamond birds. Stanwyck loved it; so did I. When we ran the test, several executives suggested that, wonderful as it was, it would look even better without the birds.

"If the birds go, the dress goes," Stanwyck said firmly. "I like 'em; so does Edith."

Rather than spend the money to make an entirely new dress . . .

The format we worked out for her was always tailored — my first evening suits, very simple, in richly embroidered fabrics. For *Sorry, Wrong Number* she wore a tailored nightgown and bed jacket. To indicate her wealth and elegance, we arranged with a Beverly Hills jeweler to lend her a fortune in gems. In addition to full insurance coverage, he insisted upon an armed guard to accompany her at all times. As small Barbara walked off the set — even when her destination was the powder room — she was shadowed instantly by a large man with two guns. A very impressive gentleman, as Barbara said, "At least they picked a good-looking one."

The only argument we ever had concerned wardrobe tests. The average female showing clothes just automatically *models*, puts one hand on her hip and walks thus . . . She'll turn her best angle to the director and the cameraman. Barbara puts on a beguiling costume and just stands before the camera, turns around, walks. I'd gesture wildly from behind the camera.

"Hand on the hip, Barbara. Come on, girl . . ."

Barbara'd have none of it. "I'm not a model, why should I act like one?" she'd say. Once a costume was in action, an actual scene being shot, the clothes became part of her characterization.

The same with Judith Anderson. Judith Anderson can look a hundred different ways — she can look dreadful or beautiful, radiant or pathetic — she's what I call a true "clothes chameleon," she can translate herself into anything. A little woman, not much taller than I, she can indicate regal height if need be. Like other top actresses from the theater, she isn't interested in her personal likes or dislikes but in whether clothes are right for the part. She is a vibrant, high-keyed woman, dynamic. I'd like someday to have her in a picture where I could do really dramatic clothes.

Loretta Young is another story. Here is a girl with whom you have only one trouble — she looks too beautiful, too elegant, and it's almost impossible to make her look anything else. She wears clothes so well that they're likely to overpower the story. "Gretchen," I call her, for I've known her since she was "Gretchen," a slender fourteen-year-old girl in *The Crusades*. The beauty was there then, and the promise, and the enthusiasm she still carries with her, there's nothing like a Loretta Young fitting.

Some actresses don't wish to see anything but the finished product. Some get confused if you show them fabrics. Some like to see just one sketch, one fabric, etc. Loretta wants to see everything, and I "rig the stage" until the Clinic looks like the *Arabian Nights*. There are bolts of all the most magnificent materials; the spotlights are on; Loretta stands before the mirrors trying each fabric while we discuss them.

Clothes are her passion; she handles herself like a model, and you know that whatever you put on her will be seen and noticed. For *The Perfect Marriage* she played a fashion magazine editor named "Maggie" who finds she and her husband, played by David Niven, are drifting apart after ten years of marriage. She determines to bring him back, and the clothes to turn the trick could be dazzling. There was a skirt of slim white jersey with a huge overskirt embroidered in gold and silver paillettes in a paisley pattern. The overskirt doubled as a cape. This I still use repeatedly at fashion shows, as I do many of the "Loretta Young" dresses. There was a white suède cloth sleeveless jacket embroidered all over with the name "Maggie" in gold. This was widely copied commercially, using cotton, wool or silk braid, rickrack or colored string for the name. The "Maggie" nightgown made the cover of *Life,* and for *Life's* inside layout I designed a gown for each of ten anniversaries, all modeled by Loretta, of course.

Loretta is not two people, she is always the same; her elegance on screen merely reflects her elegance at home. We used to have "clothes clinics" at her house, sitting in her dressing room, going over her entire wardrobe. She plans clothes long in advance. "This year I'm going to be very feminine and wear frothy clothes" . . . "This is my suit year, Edith. What do you think of this as the basis?"

Gretchen looks fragile, but when she's talking clothes she can outlast me. For that matter, she can outlast anyone on anything; behind that femininity is a will of steel. Once I got in the middle of a slight difference of opinion between her and her producer. It concerned ten gold chains she had selected to wear around the neck of a basic black dress. They looked very smart, but the producer said:

"*One* gold chain, Edith; please tell her."

"All the gold chains," Loretta told me.

"Please tell Loretta one gold chain is enough."

"But I like all the gold chains. . . ."

"One," said the producer. "You're the designer, tell her, Edith."

So Loretta wore ten gold chains. We shortened them a trifle by way of compromise.

Usually, she found a charming way of avoiding unpleasantness. If there were troubles, she said, "Edith, don't worry. We'll just call my agent." The agent handled any dirty work while Gretchen and I had the fun — up to our elbows in the very stuff of fashion, talking a language we both understand.

Ilka Chase speaks the language, too. One of the best dressed of women, Ilka was literally raised in the lap of *Vogue* (her mother was its long-time editor); and I felt considerable apprehension when she came West to make two pictures, New York is not always charitable to West Coast designers. To my great joy, she thought Hollywood was fun, and she had a true zest for clothes (and everything else). In both pictures, she played a well-dressed sophisticated career woman, herself.

When a script called for her to commute constantly between East Coast and West, I designed a twin lapel watch to fasten into the buttonholes of her lapel, one to show New York time, one Los Angeles time. We concentrated on dressmaker suits and, as "Anatole" would say, they reeked of chic. Ilka's style is so definite, I merely designed for her. If I'd had to make her into another character, it probably wouldn't have been so easy.

Ingrid Bergman I had to dress first as a nun. The picture was *The Bells of St. Mary,* and the prescription was fairly simple. I visited the Mother Superior at Immaculate Heart and worked out a costume satisfactory to the Church, but not a replica of any order. A nun's habit is slightly frustrating to a designer, and I was aching to *design,* but Bergman was perfectly happy. When we met she was wearing flat heels, no make-up, a monotone sweater and skirt, and she looked just fine. Luckily, our next picture, *Notorious,* called for high style and I had a chance to experiment. Ingrid is not a small woman; she was the tallest patient I'd ever had and not the usual clotheshorse; but she has such bearing and carriage it doesn't matter that she isn't the skinny model of the fashion magazine. Men notice clothes on a woman like this more than they do on the fashion models — she makes what she wears come to life. Some women need accessories: jewels, furs, extreme hats, feathers; the simpler Bergman's lines, the less ornamentation, the better. Simplification is the best medicine for making a beautiful woman more beautiful. Best example, the sculptured white jersey, almost Grecian dress she wore in this picture and in which she looked something like the Victory of Samothrace.

She loves freedom of motion, she dislikes high color, and that's about all I can tell you *in re* her taste. Her response to clothes? Talking about other things. She's a woman with interest in art and literature, and, except for the moments when she's before the camera, she is not an actress, not a star, no trace of pyrotechnics.

In New York, with most actresses, you shop. With Bergman, I did shop once, to find a hat we needed for picture purposes; but she's shy — she hates being stared at, and she doesn't like staring at herself; she'd rather have been in an art gallery, and the next day we went to one, to see an exhibit of scenes from famous plays in miniature, dolls taking the place of actors. This she enjoyed with her spontaneous child-like interest. When I think of Bergman I think of her at a time like that, with her happy voice, her infectious laugh. There's a calmness about her, an assurance, and an incredible optimism. She is very gay, almost naive.

And I think of her teaching me to jitterbug. We were guests at a beach house; we were listening to music and talking about dancing; I said jitterbugging looked difficult.

"You don't know how?" asked Ingrid, and promptly proceeded to teach me.

The greater the actress's background, the easier she is to work with. One of the compensations of my particular practice is meeting actresses with background; another compensation is meeting certain great ladies. Ethel Barrymore, for example. I wasn't nervous, but I was careful approaching Miss Barrymore. I needn't have been. She has the greatest charm, and a warmth to match it.

"I'm so pleased you're going to do my clothes," she said. "How do you see the picture?"

I had sketched the character in several ways (headmistress of a select finishing school in *Just For You*). Without the slightest hesitance, Miss Barrymore selected. "This is the way I should look, this is the length I wear my skirts, this is the neckline I prefer; I couldn't be more pleased." She has worked out a format for herself, even her hair style suggests the classic head of Ethel Barrymore on stage. Certain women have this perfectly worked-out format. Queen Mary of England had it; tennis star Suzanne Lenglen had it; Greta Garbo has it, and Ethel Barrymore. To women of this surety, fashion is amusing — they know what it is, but they needn't follow its whims. Miss Barrymore keeps her waistline at her waist; she always has. I felt it an honor and a privilege to dress her; we chatted about the theater and I was fascinated by her extraordinary face and voice. And do you know, I couldn't possibly tell you what she herself wore, or, for that matter, what clothes I designed for her? It didn't matter.

But in 1948 costumes mattered. That year, designers were first given recognition by the Academy of Arts and Sciences, and I had high hopes for a picture called *The Emperor Waltz*.

I can tell you every detail of every costume for that one! The picture was set in the time of Franz Joseph (1904), an era of feminine, perfectly bewitching clothes. Everything a lady wore emphasized that a lady was a lady. It was a beau-catching fashion, off-shoulder necklines exposing the round of the shoulder, tiny waists, the rose tucked in the bosom, the parasol, the fan, the veiled hat; from skin out, emphasis on provocation. No one could have worn the costumes for this princess with more finesse than Joan Fontaine, who always looks so princess and so proper and who can, on occasion, surprise you with her change of pace.

"Would you like a cup of tea?" I asked one day when she arrived, breathless, for a fitting.

"I'd like a glass of cold champagne!" she said, and promptly had an ice bucket and the wine brought up from her car.

I'd worked with Joan before; I knew how well she'd wear these hourglass styles, and I wasn't disappointed. Sure of myself I'd never been; but seeing the daily rushes, I *knew*: these were the loveliest clothes I'd ever seen. They would certainly win the Academy Award. What could possibly be better?

For myself, for the great night of the Awards, I had a dress of black, embroidered in gold and silver, high-necked, with long panels of the same Oriental embroidery. The motif of the design: tiny elephants whose trunks turned up, a sign of good luck. I couldn't lose.

The award went to *Joan of Arc*. I've never been sure of anything since.

Actually, the basis for the Academy Award is not how beautiful the costumes are but how much they contribute to the picture, how integral a part they are of telling the story. I won my first award the following year, with *The Heiress*. The costumes were not pretty; the problem was to make Olivia de Havilland *un*attractive. The fabrics were harsh serge, stiff wools, uncompromising as to color, severe as to neckline. I dressed Olivia as a mature woman rather than as the girl she was, and placed her against a background of women who looked young and gay. At the dance, where the others wore tulle and organdy, she wore dark, heavy silk embroidered in jet. Then, toward the end of the picture, when she wished to get revenge on Montgomery Clift, allure him, we made a complete transition into softer, more feminine colors and fabrics.

Let me also add that every detail of these costumes was correct down to the last buttonhole. Olivia not only joined me in the research, she initiated some of it. We visited museums in New York together, studying original petticoats and corsets of the period; we read Henry James's *Washington Square*, on which the script was based. Olivia would come flying in with a wonderful scoop, some detail of lingerie, some way of fixing her hair, all absolutely authentic. At fittings she tried out the motions of walking, sitting, dancing. Costumes of this period (mid-nineteenth century) are treacherous, because of the understructure — the pantalets, corset covers, hoops — and because of the width of the skirts. Dedicated and thoroughgoing as she is, Olivia worked out the mechanics and wore her clothes with grace.

In the same picture, Miriam Hopkins, fresh from sables and diamonds on stage in New York, was cast as Olivia's aunt. Not just an aunt, but a poor aunt. Not just a poor aunt, but a widow. Up to my ears in accuracy as I was, Miriam almost seduced me. "In those days any woman could be attractive," Miriam said sagely, "no matter how poor. She could use an enchanting little lace collar and cuffs — why, this is the kind of woman who would while away the hours making little lace cuffs! Wouldn't she, Edith?"

Now I have a great respect for stage actresses. I know that to them reality is a religion, so . . . But when we were finally ready to show the costumes to Willie Wyler, I had misgivings. Miriam looked as little like someone's aunt as possible, and not in the least impoverished. Mr. Wyler circled her like a prospective buyer. "I don't feel we quite have the character," said he, and left the room. The "poor" aunt's costumes were done over, and with the same flawless respect for history and personality we'd used on the niece.

After all the liberties we'd taken in the days of ermine-trimmed bathrobes and décolletage westerns, *The Heiress* was good for my schoolteacher soul. It certainly was the best job of costuming I'd ever done, and it won an Oscar. This time I wasn't excited, and I didn't dress up. Oscar was a year late. But he *was* golden, and he never turned black like my silver loving cup.

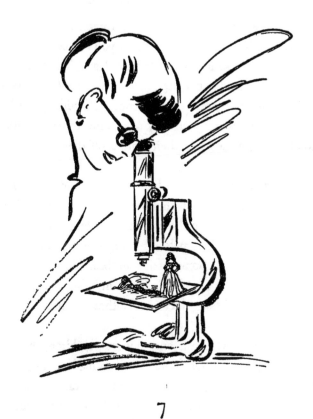

7

The Doctor Looks at Life

ACTRESSES HAVE LITTLE in common. They are as diversified as women in any walk of life, and, as women in any walk of life, their motives, manners and goals differ widely. Every cultured, charming star with whom you work gives you something. But you learn, too, from the less talented, the ambition-driven, the would-bes. They are all human beings — though you may doubt it on a bad day when you've been coping with one of the breed so in love with herself and her looks that no designer can handle her, one who usually affects the spectacular, out-of-this-world clothes associated with "*gone* Hollywood." Each has her own way of coming to terms with life; and often when they take their clothes off they take their hair down.

I've observed the careers of happy women and tragic women, some so timid they put on their costumes alone behind closed doors, some delighted to show their black lace panties studded with diamonds or their pale pink lingerie embroidered with well-known names. Some arrive in best bib and tucker to impress me — "Just a tired old Balmain," they'll sigh. Others effect the most casual of casual clothes to show how little impressed *they* are.

I've had brothers, aunts and mothers, children, uncles and lovers brought to fittings. Some of them made an appreciative audience, some thought I didn't know fashion from a hole in the ground — and if there's anything I do know, after living in mining camps all my childhood, it's a *hole* in the ground. Some of them gave me helpful hints — no extra charge. I've also played host to tigers, baby elephants, cats and dogs. Jean Wallace brought along her parrot Louis to see how he'd go with her gown, since the bird's appearing with her in the picture. Louis behaved a good deal better than some of the children who've been raised by progressive methods — if the little darlings want to eat a pin . . .

No two fittings are alike. Dietrich never stops to rest. Hedy Lamarr spent a good part of each fitting on the horizontal. Under my spotlights in a slinky, gold-beaded gown, she'd look like the all-time *femme fatale*. Then, suddenly, she'd turn those great translucent eyes on me and say, "Edith, I must rest. When you have had children, you have backaches." And, half-finished though we were, down she'd lie. When she didn't like a dress, she'd lie down even oftener. She ate constantly. A Hedy Lamarr fitting meant food shuttled in every hour or so, Viennese pastries, pot-roast sandwiches, anything to eat; and, while she rested, the sultry, exotic temptress munched and talked of her three children.

Hedy is the most unself-conscious siren ever born. She's as relaxed and boneless as a Persian cat; she has no temper, she likes to wear dirndls and simple blouses; she has never been even momentarily confused between self and symbol. She knows what she looks like, but she doesn't work at it; and this ability of hers for relaxation means she'll never have a wrinkle or a bulge.

Typical Hedy Lamarr clothes are slinky black with pearls, slinky beaded gowns, slinky chiffon peignoirs. What she designs for herself — and she loves designing her own personal clothes — neither slinks nor slithers. Even in her screen clothes, there was a point where she'd draw the line. For *Samson and Delilah*, we had sketched costumes with a voluptuous bustline Hedy couldn't fill.

"I'm not a big bosomy woman," she said (she's slim actually); "if you pad me I'll look ridiculous. I won't be able to act. I'll feel as if I'm carting balloons." So her costumes were not padded; we achieved a voluptuous effect by line, by drapery, and nothing could have been lovelier than the Delilah I took to Mr. de Mille in a costume of mesh and beaten silver, so lovely he actually *smiled!* For Mr. de Mille's smile you almost forgave Hedy her predilection for the horizontal and the edible.

Hedy always thinks like a woman. Bette Davis thinks like a businessman. Hers is a truly organized point of view, and working with her I've felt like being in conference with a bank president. You can see the authority on screen in her walk, her voice, her action; there's not a trace of indecision — she's the same on screen and off; and she's only one of the most sensational experiences I've ever had.

She came in like a small whirlwind, the first time. There was no polite chitchat. She's a busy woman, I'm a busy woman, and we both knew it was a nice day. She'd come, actually, to see if we had the same point of view.

"This is how I walk," she said (it's a walk like a whiplash). "I must move freely. If clothes don't move with me, I can't wear them. This woman (in *June Bride*) is a career woman; she works for a magazine; and strangely enough she's a lot like me. How do you think she should dress?"

"Like a career woman who doesn't look like a career woman," I said, and quickly did a little sketch of a Bette Davis striding about in a coat dress with open and concealed pockets, the concealed pockets for pencils, memo pads, etc.

"A high-fashion carpenter's coverall!" She grinned a regular blockbuster of a grin, and we were in business. Bette liked the coat dress so much she had six of them made for herself in varied colors. She was wearing one the day we started working on *All About Eve*. She strode about, hands deep in her pockets, studying the fabrics, the sketches. For each costume, I'd place my favorite sketch on top, then alternates. In nothing flat, she'd whipped around the room, selected each of the top drawings, and was saying, "When do we fit?"

This is never a tense or dramatic woman, it's a woman terribly interested in whatever she's doing and doing it with tremendous energy, and enthusiasm . . . a brilliant woman, who enters into a story conference less like the star than like the director, her concern with the whole not with herself . . . an impatient woman who has none of the usual female vanity, she never thinks, Do I look nice in this? She thinks only, Is it good for the part? . . . A small woman, not thin, she can look tall, regal, short, chic or slovenly, whatever is needed for a scene, and each scene is played to the hilt.

Up here in the Clinic, Bette "does" the entire picture. Each dress has to be tried for all the action the scene will demand: the taffeta dress for the drunk scene, the suit (with its tight skirt) for the scene where she throws herself across the bed. Unfortunately there was no bed. That didn't deter Bette. She seized my two big ottomans, pushed them against the couch, took a running leap, dropped her mink (no one can drop a mink more elegantly) and threw herself! The skirt held together!

"Guess it'll work," she said.

All About Eve was an exciting picture from the beginning. You smell smoke when there's a good fire and this was good. Bette's take-off on a successful New York actress showed her at the top of her form: no accident could throw her; any fault — in costume, dialogue, or what have you — immediately became in her hands an asset. When we tested the brown taffeta dress trimmed in sable for the party sequence, the dress slipped repeatedly off her shoulder. What to do? Could we use tape? A net yoke? Elastic around the neckline? Bette shrugged and it promptly slipped off her shoulder again.

"Why not let it?" she said. The dress was moving with her, it was right.

We had lunch one day after the picture had become a success and I'd won an award for the costumes. We talked about businesswomen not being very feminine. It isn't true, of course.

"You can't fool me, Edith," Bette said. "You may live with potted cactuses but you love hearts and flowers." And the next day she sent me a great flowered heart.

The career girl who *doesn't* live with potted cactuses is Jennifer Jones. Where Bette Davis enters like a whirlwind, Jennifer glides in like a gentle breeze. She's a calm, romantic girl who has developed an individual style of her own — poetic, charming, almost Victorian. I think of her always carrying a sable muff with a bunch of fresh violets in it. She loves pretty clothes and they suit her. She's one of the few in pictures who can wear period clothes without making them look like costumes (in *Sister Carrie*, for example). When I first had her in *Love Letters*, I found her a sensitive and interested patient. She was to play a girl who had lost her memory, and we tried soft, fragile wools to establish the mood. Many stars have first and last say on costumes; but Jennifer prefers having her director or producer make decisions. She gets things done by a charming, passive feminine approach.

In *Love Letters*, Hal Wallis thought the wedding dress too conventional, too pretty — not in the right mood for the story. It happened to be the dress Jennifer and I liked best, and I was upset. In this instance, the patient soothed the doctor.

"Never mind, Edith, we'll use it somehow, someday."

Jennifer must have confidence in the people with whom she works, once she's sure. . . . I've been called in several emergencies. Once, in the middle of the night, David Selznick phoned me. An important scene for his *Ruby Gentry* was to be shot next day, and Jennifer had broken her finger. It wasn't the pain that was bothering her, but worry over how the broken finger might be concealed. The "cure" was a special cuff that would fasten to the splint and a huge ring to fit over the splint. It didn't interfere in the least, it even added a little to the Victorian charm. Another emergency concerned her last-minute replacement of Elizabeth Taylor for the Academy Award presentation. She described by phone what she had, and I suggested a pearl-white, delicately embroidered gown in the romantic mood that is Jennifer's key.

A key is what each woman must have, and no one ever had it more superbly than Gloria Swanson. It's been a long time since she drove up with her Marquis and we threw roses; but Gloria today is still Gloria — a star, a fashion plate.

Can you imagine what a thrill it was for me to do *Sunset Boulevard?* Trouble, too; for in this picture Gloria was to look like an actress who has passed her peak, a star in the discard, living on memories. I based the clothes on what she had worn in earlier days. (We used the very same shoes. She wears a size 2½; you can't buy that size in Los Angeles today, but in Wardrobe we found size 2½'s with Gloria's name on them, shoes she'd worn twenty years before.) We made the tests; went to a projection room to view them; and what happened was utter consternation. Because of her bone structure and assurance, Miss Swanson projected on screen just about as she had twenty years before. She walked on in a pair of tight jersey hostess pajamas with an overskirt of leopardskin — and there she was, not in the least like a has-been.

There was very little I could do about the clothes to accomplish the effect needed. It had to be done with make-up and lighting; because, no matter what you put on this woman, she walks with the air of a woman who knows she's glamorous. This is no actress who's just discovered a format; this is an actress who has been herself so long — first of the four-star stars — that she's used to herself and stardom is as natural as breathing.

You pay her homage because she *is* this, and because she's the living example of what she preaches: that clothes are supremely important, that a woman must never be caught any time or any place looking less than she should. If today's stars sometimes run out to shop or to the studio in blue jeans or in a sweater that's seen better days, this lady does not. She is meticulously groomed, whether in black jersey smothered in black fox or in a dark grey wool dress with small black hat, bag, gloves and shoes. She wears hats with everything except her nightgowns. If you drop in at her house unexpectedly, you'll find her in smart slacks, her hair up in a turban, looking completely assembled, completely like a motion picture star. She's small and likes to emphasize that smallness; so, even when a shoulder-length mane of hair was popular, she kept her small look by wearing a bandeau or a turban, keeping her hair close and neat. She never allows color to overpower her either, staying with black, gray, brown and beige. She has an unusual face; why not let people see it without being distracted by the color of her gloves?

Gloria is a woman of the world who has lived in all the great capitals, makes many TV appearances, and is interested in many things; whatever interests her she wants to interest her friends as well. Recently she visited me and talked of world politics. Women are *important* to politics, she was saying; professional women who have so much to contribute should not be engrossed in their own profession to the exclusion of international affairs. I haven't found out yet what she has in mind for me to do in politics, but *I will*.

What she has in mind for me in terms of reforming my food habits I already know. Gloria is a devotee of brewer's yeast, whole-grain health bread and organically grown vegetables. She feels that you live and look according to what you eat; and I must admit that, sitting across her dinner table, observing her faultless skin, you seriously consider throwing away your lamb chop for her oats and greens.

"It will rejuvenate you, Edith," she says, handing me a gold-wrapped package that might have come from Cartier's — a loaf of her bread!

She's not the first star who has tried to teach this doctor a few new tricks. I deal with creative women, and, much as they revere my advice, they're sure I'm a babe in the woods so far as my *self* is concerned. Mary Martin tried to fix my hair; Clara Bow wanted to give me a waistline; from Loretta Young to Carolyn Jones, they've tried to change the spots — but no one ever had more plans for me than Jane Wyman. She's a changer by nature, a very definite girl, a perfectionist, and not one bit intimidated by my venerable status.

"I think I'll have roast beef," I may say, glancing at a menu.

"Are you out of your mind?" cries Jane. "You can have that any time; let's have something deadly and wonderful — the cold salmon with cucumbers vinaigrette. You spend too much time, Edith, eating what you think is good for you. Listen to Mother."

One day we were having steaks and Jane ordered hers with chopped onion on the side. Mine came the same way, and she noticed that I was eschewing the onions.

"Why don't you eat your onions?"

"They make me ill."

"That's *all* in your mind," cried Jane.

So I ate them. "How do you feel?" she asked, phoning me during the afternoon.

"Ill," I said, and was.

Jane is a gay girl, and I like her. When she came to me for *Here Comes the Groom* and for *Just for You,* she was fresh from a series of heavy dramas; she hadn't been thinking in high-fashion terms, and it was my turn to say, "Now listen to Mother. . . ." Actually, Jane is a type. She is very young in appearance, very pert, and in personality not at all the heavy dramatic girl. She has none of the star complex, but she does have a definite idea of what she can and cannot wear. She prefers simple clothes, but when she wears high fashion she wears it — to the teeth.

Jane isn't about to agree with anything you tell her; but you can always argue. Sometimes she wins, sometimes I do. In *Just For You*, we needed a theatrical costume and I had sketched a black net number with black net hose.

Jane took a quick look. "I can't *wear* anything that short, Edith."

"Why not?"

"I'm not a pin-up girl."

"You have beautiful legs."

"It'll have to be longer."

So we made it, fit it and even Jane had to admit that if she's not a pin-up, she'll have to do till a pin-up comes along. As a matter of fact, we finally made it even shorter than the sketch had suggested.

For her personal wardrobe and for the screen, I like Jane in very tailored clothes. Her face is so unusual you don't want frills or fluff or extreme styles to distract from that face or from the charming abruptness of motion that is uniquely hers.

The greatest brain storm Janie ever had in my behalf was when we were making *Lucy Gallant.* In it she was to play the very chic owner of a dress salon. The action of the picture included a fashion show, and Janie decided that no one should commentate that fashion show but me.

"It's type casting," she said.

"I'm not an actress!"

"I'll coach you; it'll be a breeze."

"What should I wear?" I said.

"A traditional suit. Don't worry about a thing. Now listen to Mother. . . ."

The next thing I knew, I was cast as Edith Head in *Lucy Gallant* and was studying my script. Now, I've been on radio and television, I've taught school, I've lectured to women's clubs and commentated numerous fashion shows. This wasn't going to throw *me.* But as zero hour approached, I found myself running around muttering my lines like crazy. The director and producer had decided that I should appear without my glasses; that the audience reaction to them on screen would be: "Dark glasses! Hollywood affectation."

On the fatal day, I reported as per call, in make-up, at 7 A.M. My hair was done; my face was done; Jane had had a smock made with my name on it — that cheered me somewhat; but now that I was made-up, they wouldn't let me put on my glasses for fear of smearing. I wandered about in a fog, hunting for the sound stage. When I finally did find it, I discovered that Jane had arranged my dressing room right next to hers and that my name and a small star were in evidence on the dressing-room door. At nine, I was ready and waiting; but nine, ten, eleven and twelve came and went and the fashion show hadn't been called — or me.

"Come on, I'll take you to lunch," Jane said. "We'll run through your lines."

"Please," I said, "I've got to put my glasses on; I can't stand it a minute longer."

We wrapped my frames in cotton and at least I could see; but when I ran through my lines, Janie was horrified. So were Thelma Ritter, Claire Trevor, Charlton Heston.

"Edith, you're mumbling!" Jane said. The others nodded corroboration.

"Thank you, it's such a pleasure to be here and meet the governor," I mumbled over and over while they ate. *I couldn't* eat, I couldn't swallow. I could only say, "Thank you, it's such a pleasure . . ."

We got back to the set at one o'clock. Work went on. One, two, three, four, five . . . I was still rehearsing my lines. I was almost frantic. I'd never realized acting was such a difficult business. Finally, at a quarter past five, I was called for my "big dramatic scene." The models were lined up, the fashion show started, and I stood there commenting on clothes, as I've done hundreds of times — only this was different. This time there was a camera looking at me, and I couldn't see it. Without my glasses, I couldn't see much of anything.

"Look this way." . . . "Pull in your tummy." . . . "Don't duck your head." . . . "Camera." . . . "Action." . . .

I'll tell you frankly, it was the worst day of my life. I did the scene; I saw the rushes; I promptly gave up acting. And I've had a slightly higher regard for all my lovely guinea pigs ever since.

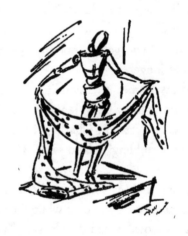

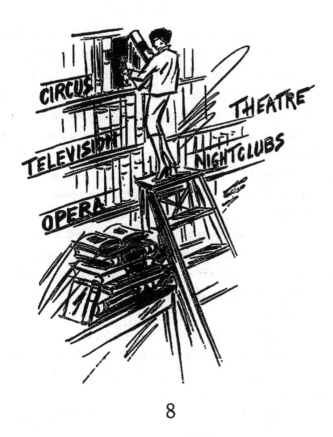

8

From Circus to Grand Opera

MY PRACTICE isn't limited to motion picture problems. I've designed costumes for circus and opera, for television, for Las Vegas, for nightclub and benefit appearances, even for governors' inaugurations. Can't you just see Hedy Lamarr sitting atop an elephant the night of St. John's circus benefit, dressed elegantly in chiffon trousers and a few well-chosen beads? Or Barbara Stanwyck, in velvet riding habit and plumed hat, riding a trained horse side-saddle around the ring? Or Effie Klinker taking to television with Edgar Bergen in an original jumper? Or Marialice Shivers wearing a gown of mother-of-pearl lace for her husband's second inauguration as Governor of Texas? (The gown was copied from one we'd used in a fashion show in *Lucy Gallant*. Governor Shivers, playing himself in that picture, had asked that if he were re-elected, would I copy that dress for his wife? He was, and I did.)

My patients lead pretty dynamic lives and their clothes personalities go with them. One recent assignment: Freddie Brisson's Broadway production, *The Pleasure of His Company*, which gave me a chance to work again with Cornelia Otis Skinner.

We worked together first on the movie, *Our Hearts Were Young and Gay*, when Cornelia came out not as an actress, but as co-author and technical advisor with Emily Kimbrough. Theirs was a story of their own youth in the 20's, when as flappers they went on their great pilgrimmage to Paris. I'd been through the flapper era with Clara Bow, but Cornelia and Emily didn't know that; besides, theirs was a different kind of flapper — guileless girls searching for glamour. In Paris they spent all their precious money for white fox coats that promptly disintegrated. We had some very gay consultations and hoped someday we'd have a chance to do a picture with more exciting clothes. Then I had Cornelia for *The Uninvited* with Ray Milland. This time she was the actress, but with just one costume change; so again we said, "Some-day . . ."

Then it happened. In *The Pleasure of His Company* she plays a smart, well-dressed modern woman, a successful woman, not unlike herself. Perhaps the clothes are a shade higher key than Cornelia actually wears — she has so many alter egos on stage, she can be a trifle more conservative in person. For the stage, however, she feels, "The audience must know who *she* is the moment she walks on. They make instant judgment before they've even heard her speak; and they resent deeply being deceived. She can't look like one thing and be another."

Since the first scene is spring in San Francisco, Miss Skinner appears in a gray suit lined with gray-and-white print, with a matching print blouse, white hat, the whitest pearls and gloves. With her own vivid coloring and brown eyes, she conveys positive health, alertness and vitality. She's a woman with a grown daughter; her husband still loves her, and she's interested in how she looks. In the same scene, incidentally, Dolores Hart, playing the daughter about to be married, wears a soft suit, in taste similar enough to her "mother's" that "mother" might have selected it.

The mother's clothes and the daughter's clothes aren't competitive because actually there's no *age* in clothes today. You don't go in and buy "one suit for a woman of forty-five, please." It's the personality and the figure that count. For Cornelia Otis Skinner, I planned the same type of clothes I wear myself: smart, simple, no frippery. She is a tall woman and I'm a small one, but we have the same point of view: we wouldn't be caught dead in a pinafore, we find being adult an exciting thing.

"Isn't it wonderful?" Cornelia says. "By the time you're adult you've found out what you can and cannot do, you don't try to do things that play against you. You stay within the frame of your own capacity, just as you stay within a character on stage. You don't try a character you can't believe or that the audience won't believe; you shouldn't in real life either."

Those of you who've seen her on stage in *The Pleasure of His Company* found her believable, I'm sure, adult and fresh in her black chiffon, her Oriental silk hostess gown, her mossy green day dress. Clothes for the theater differ from movie clothes because detail matters less and the total effect, full length, is always *on*. I went to New Haven for the tryout and was as jittery as if this were my professional debut.

Another recent departure, the record album "Lizabeth," Lizabeth Scott singing. For the album photo in full color, Scott asked me to do a dress that would capture the effect we'd achieved once in a picture where she played a nightclub singer. "I'm not a nightclub singer, never was; the dress gave me the armor that made me feel safe in the role," she said. Confronted with the record album, she wanted the same look and the same feel. Now, most nightclub singers are arrayed in glitter; they're underdressed and sheathed so tightly every high note threatens to burst the whole. For Scott I used no glitter, no tightness. The clinging look was accomplished with

cool blue jersey, dramatically simple. Scott is herself dramatically simple, and she plays parts much like herself. She
dresses the same for her roles as for real life.

So does Anne Baxter. I've designed for Anne for more than
ten years; she was one patient who had worked out her own
format before she ever arrived at the Clinic; not a patient —
a collaborator, wanting not help but new fashion. She is a
girl with many interests; she's smart, sophisticated, and loves
sophisticated clothes. So you can imagine how frustrated
we both were when she was cast in *The Ten Commandments*
as the Egyptian princess, Nefertiri. I'd been doing research
on this picture for years; I was completely aware of Nefertiri
and her sinister, hawklike brooding face, the face of a lady
vulture. And then in walked Anne, with her pert Irish look
and tilted nose! We both suffered over that one, but *The
Ten Commandments* has made nothing but money; no critic
has said a word against Irish Anne as the Egyptian —where
does that leave us? Suffice it to say, we've had a good deal
more fun designing clothes recently for Anne's TV appearances where her very definite personality can be very definitely
enhanced.

My first exciting brush with television was when NBC
opened its big studio in the San Fernando Valley and Roz
Russell was mistress of ceremonies. She wanted to look like
"a famous MC" and she knew I'd done work for television
before; so in she came to the Clinic and we worked out a
happy diagnosis. Roz is a great clotheshorse. She has a
model's figure, a model's assurance, plus a gay, vivid per-

sonality; I "did" her in charcoal chiffon with flat sequins. It photographed black.

The chief difference, incidentally, between designing for television and for movies is a matter of lighting. On a television set, you have overhead lighting. On live TV you don't change the lighting for close, medium or long shots; your colors must be less subtle, more definite. In making movies, you camera-test all wardrobe before it is used. There's no time for this on TV. In movies, you also see daily rushes. But here we were going on before an audience of forty million with no preview, and you play it safe. For black: dark blue or charcoal; for white: light blue, pale gray or off-white. I never use *color* per se, what I want on screen is black, white or gray.

Roz's dress was very slim, long-sleeved, low-necked — now for some attention-getters to add drama. We tried a short stole, a long stole, a fur cape. They weren't dramatic enough.

"What would people least expect me to wear?" Roz said.

"The world's largest muff." And I sketched one promptly, a gigantic black fox muff. "Also a small black feather hat."

A few days later, she stood under my spotlights trying on hat after hat. We'd gone to Rex, selected dozens, and now were trying for the total look. Roz would put on a hat, take up her muff and pantomine the world's idea of a movie star.

"Too, too beautiful!" . . . "Too, too sweet!" . . . "Too, too chic!" . . . Roz would say, making hilarious fun of herself. "How can I look smart, Edith, without frightening people? Without looking like a caricature?"

We ended up selecting a small explosion of black feathers; Roz batted her eyelashes, laughed, and agreed it was right, it was smart, it wouldn't frighten them (too high fashion frightens some people).

In designing for nightclubs, as differentiated from television or movies, there is the difference again in lighting. You must be careful not to select a color that will turn pea-green when hit by an amber spot, and the effect of your clothes is always full length rather than close up. That's why I went to Las Vegas when I designed nightclub clothes for Betty Hutton and subsequently for Rosemary Clooney. Rosemary is another girl who first came to me with white fluffy dresses, full skirts, little waists, bows on the shoes — the young girl look. She was well dressed and expensively dressed, but she hadn't jelled. She flitted from dress to dress with equal enthusiasm; and the very fact that people call her "Rosie," that she is a natural blonde with curly hair, then a singer with a band, led her to favor very feminine girlish styles.

For this same Rosie we worked out practically a uniform; suits, sports dresses, dinner clothes, formal clothes, always the same short length (which suits her proportions) with emphasis on the collar and neckline. The clothes are simple, sophisticated, of plain fabric and color, because essentially you don't notice what this girl wears, you notice her vitality. From the beginning, Rosemary's attitude was: "If Joe likes it, I do." And I *knew* José Ferrer'd like it; I'd checked him first.

This is what you call "making a clothes personality"; we

experimented first with various necklines, various silhouettes; I even had Rosie come into the gallery and we photographed her in our experiments. (If they would photograph women in department stores, and the "patient" could see the picture, she'd often say, "Oh, NO!" Frequently, when you look only in the mirror, you see just what you wish to see — say, from the waist up.) From the beginning, Rosemary was an interested patient and one who took the medicine prescribed.

I've known her and designed for her on three different levels: for pictures, for nightclub engagements, and for the pregnant woman who wants to be smart and pretty. She's been pregnant four times in almost as many years, and Rosemary's not the kind of girl who can just retire and look enceinte. She works in television and nightclubs, she travels with José all over the world, and, several pregnancies ago, she called me:

"Edith, we're leaving for London next week. We're going to meet interesting people and go to many interesting places. I can't get into a thing, and Joe is such a snob about clothes!"

He is; and Rosemary dresses *for* him. I designed for her a series of full-length coats with deep inverted pleats and a Clooney collar. We've had these made in every color and fabric from black taffeta to beige linen. This last time they were no longer recognized as maternity clothes, they were the same shape as the then popular trapeze.

Rosemary keeps coming back; many of my patients do — that's what's so pleasant. What is frustrating is not to get a

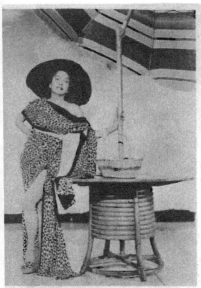

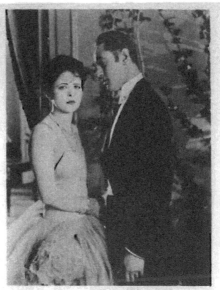

's been a long time since she drove
p and we threw roses; but Gloria
wanson today is still Gloria, a star.
(*In* Sunset Boulevard)

Clara Bow wanted to look young,
sexy, the symbol of Flaming Youth.
She was selling on the screen what
she was — a glamorous Flapper.

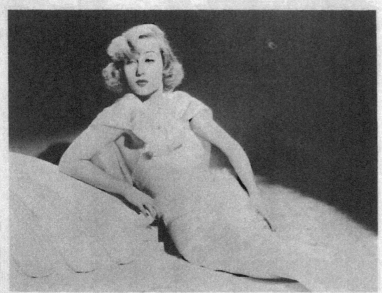

Carole Lombard loved tailored clothes, she hated clothes that looked,
she said, "like a cross between French pastry and a lampshade."

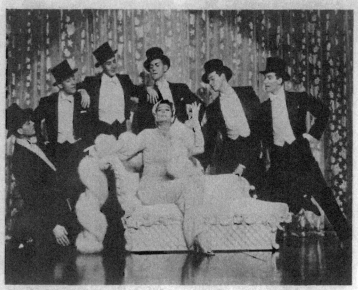

Rosalind Russell is a great clothes personality. She would put on a hat, and pantomime the world's idea of a movie star.
(*In* THE GIRL RUSH)

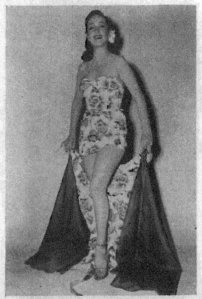

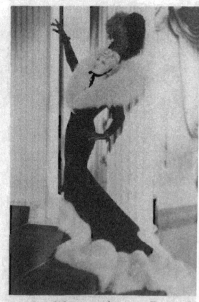

Dorothy and her silk sarong became the household Polynesian.

Mae West taught me all that I know about sex — clotheswise. "I like 'em tight, girls," she said.

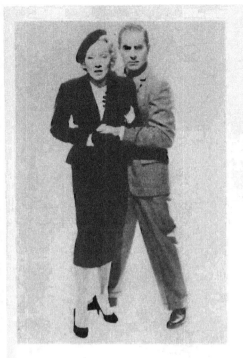

Fashion is a language. Some know it, some learn it, some never will. But Dietrich was born knowing. She looks like all the fashion magazine covers rolled into one.

(*With Tyrone Power in* Witness for the Prosecution)

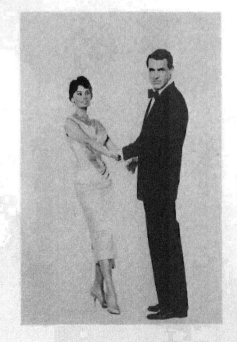

I consider Cary Grant the most beautifully dressed man in the world. "I do not wear blue jeans," said Sophia Loren in her beautiful English.

(*In* Houseboat)

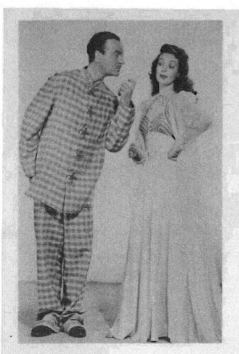

Loretta Young is a girl with whom you have only one trouble — she looks too beautiful, too elegant, and it's almost impossible to make her look anything else.
(*With David Niven*)

No one can *drop* a mink more elegantly than Bette Davis.
(*In* ALL ABOUT EVE)

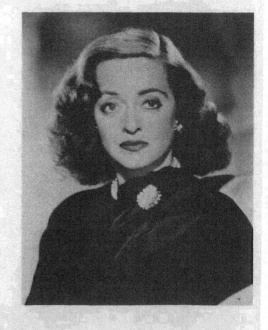

few of the patients you'd like to *have*. Deborah Kerr is one! She is a friend, and I wish we had more time together. Friendships aren't easy in Hollywood. We're all extremely busy; there isn't must time for friendship, and you're very careful where you place it. Many actresses, by the very nature of their ambition, must have a strong core of self-interest and self-concentration. Deborah has the capacity for friendship; she has intelligence, warmth; she's a real human being. And one of my tragedies! I've had her for two pictures, both "costume-less," *The Proud and the Profane*, for example, in which she played an Army nurse in an Army nurse's uniform. The one lovely gown I've ever designed for her was an aqua satin for a benefit performance, at which she was master of ceremonies. It was an impressive gown, with a full-length, exquisitely embroidered stole; it literally swept onto the stage, and Deborah adored it — until she tried to sit down. The dress wouldn't sit; she had to bring it back to the Clinic for a further operation so that it could go to the theater, etc.

Most people think of an Englishwoman as being reserved, slightly cool. Deborah is reserved in her manner; she has a dignity, but she also has such an infectious gaiety! When she comes in for a fitting, we can't wait for her to take off her clothes. Last time her underslip was embroidered in pink roses and "Spring is here." Another time, she wore a petticoat that said, "What's new?"

Another of my tragedies is Joan Crawford. I've known Joan since Clara Bow days. One of my hopes has always been,

"Someday I'm going to do a picture with her!" And then it happened. The picture was to be called *Lisbon;* Joan moved onto the lot; we sipped champagne and nibbled fresh caviar every evening in her dressing room, and went over sketches. It was the sort of assignment to dream of. Joan was playing a very, very wealthy woman, a very beautiful woman, a woman with superb taste. Our materials were ordered, the patterns were in work, the designs for jewelry sent to the jeweler, the shoes ordered, and I had caught the rare excitement you get working with a great mannequin. Then, for some reason I've never understood, *Lisbon* was called off; Miss Crawford moved off the lot. Someday I'm still going to get her — for a picture, a TV stint, or an appearance at the Academy Awards.

One of my extracurricular duties is as consultant to the Academy, and during the month of March the number of problems and diagnoses are of epidemic proportions. For instance, in 1958 Eva Marie Saint called in to say she was going to have a baby, she didn't want to have a new dress made, did I think she could get into the black velvet I'd made her for *That Certain Feeling?* We moved a few hooks and Eva Marie made one of the most successful appearances of the evening. Zsa Zsa Gabor brought in every dress she owned, tried them on; we decided against all of them. (I couldn't make her one, she wasn't under contract.) Then she phoned. "Darling, I'm in great trouble. There are three beautiful dresses at Elizabeth Arden's; I don't know which to choose."

I met her after work at Arden's. The dresses were stunning, and Zsa Zsa, perfect example of the word "female," is in her element in an evening gown. (I've never seen her in tailored clothes; she typifies extravagance, high fashion removed from reality.) My only trouble was saying *which*, and I finally decided on the pale, pale pink. On the night of the Awards, Zsa Zsa phoned me.

"Darling, I have a surprise for you. I'm not going to wear *any* of those . . ."

The Awards are important because they are viewed by such a large audience. For a designer, a large audience *is* important; it is very rewarding to have a patient like Dorothy Kirsten and to see her on the Firestone Hour on television or singing in concert at the Hollywood Bowl in creations of mine. With her glorious operatic voice, Dorothy has tried concerts and loved them — tried television, loved that — tried Las Vegas, was mad about it — still continues singing opera; and I am involved on all fronts. The *Opera News*, March 17, 1958, carried this note:

> Dorothy Kirsten, on leave from the Metropolitan this season, celebrated her 50th *Tosca* in Miami, singing four performances in eight days. Edith Head, award-winning Hollywood designer, created a new second-act gown for the diva: royal garnet velvet trimmed in diamonds and topped by a full length cape of the same material lined in gold lamé.

I used no motion picture touches on Dorothy's *Tosca* costume, I merely translated a person who is very blond to the role of a brunette. Tosca was a successful court singer, the gown could be as regal as you'd wish, the velvet would look handsome on stage and no worry about it photographing too bulky.

When you're designing operatic clothes for a movie, you

must watch the bulk (as I learned in my first tangle with opera, a Valkyrie costume for Madame Kirsten Flagstad). But when I first designed for Dorothy Kirsten, the picture was *Mr. Music* and she was playing a great prima donna *off* stage, in lovely modern clothes. Dorothy, thank heaven, is a woman who is not built like the traditional opera singer: she's a tall, beautiful blond Viking and I dress her off stage exactly as an opera singer doesn't look. She loves clothes; she has a flair for wearing them; she's an outgoing person, easy to work with — indeed, I discovered that opera has less temperament than motion pictures!

I even made her wedding dress, of palest blue-white lace, and for Las Vegas we've had a field day, with prima donna clothes that convey, we think, the popular idea of how an opera star would look. This is strictly the "first night" look: magnificent brocades, sables, jewels, lamés, velvets; and so far as the nightclub circuit is concerned, these clothes are Dorothy's signature, as white glittery jeweled gowns are Dietrich's and fresh, short young evening dresses Clooney's.

Nightclubs have become the "theater" of our day in terms of glamour, while pictures have become concerned with realism. We are now primarily in a period of personality clothes. The way an actress looks on screen or on television or on the street — much the same. For me, it's a far happier era than my apprenticeship, when I was constantly involved with the bizarre. And of course, in designing these modern personality clothes, I've worked with some of the most exciting personalities of all time.

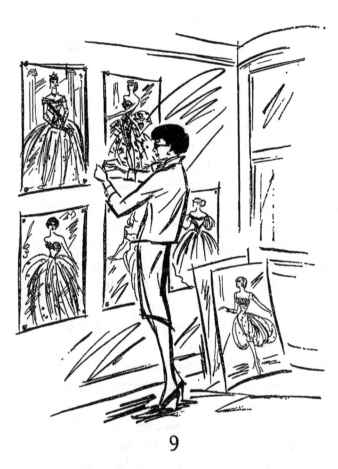

9

Glamorous Guinea Pigs

EARLY IN 1952, I hurried to New York to show sketches for the picture *Roman Holiday*. The film was to be shot in Rome, the young star was appearing on Broadway in a play called *Gigi*. She had never had a large movie role; I'd seen the test she made in Europe, but the test had been shot in pajamas and I had no idea, really, how Audrey Hepburn looked.

She came to see me wearing a little dark suit with white collars and cuffs, very simple, very elegant, with a sprig of lily-of-the-valley in her buttonhole, fresh white gloves, her whole person clean and shining — a little girl with the poise of the Duchess of Windsor. Her figure and flair told me, at once, here was a girl who'd been born to make designers happy. If she were not an actress she'd be a model or a designer. As it is, she's all three: a girl way ahead of high fashion, who deliberately looks different from other women, who has dramatized her own slenderness into her chief asset.

A good model figure is at most 34-22-34. It's a figure you seldom see in movie business. During a "bust" season, you'll have actress after actress boasting a 38 or 39; and during any season, your top dramatic stars are likely to be short and not necessarily symmetrical. Audrey has the perfect model figure: very slim and tall (5'6¾). She doesn't wear pads; she accentuates her slimness; and she has the cultivated taste so dear to a dress doctor. Audrey knows more about fashion than any actress save Dietrich. Like Dietrich, her fittings are the ten-hour not the ten-minute variety. To the sketches for *Roman Holiday*, she added a few of her own preferences: simpler necklines, wider belts. I returned to the coast, had the clothes made, and we tested them in New York. When I saw the test, I knew that this was not only a fine actress (I'd already caught *Gigi*) but one of the greatest models. The clothes translated her perfectly from a prim little princess to an eager young girl on the streets of Rome. Audrey won an Oscar for *Roman Holiday*; so did I, and I looked forward to her next picture, *Sabrina*.

Planning the clothes this time, I went up to San Francisco where she was playing on stage. I took with me pages and pages of "little Audreys" — the Hepburn face and figure in miniature, on which Audrey could doodle dresses. She loves to design, and we worked like a team on the *Sabrina* clothes, in which the chauffeur's daughter goes to Europe and comes back *très chic*. The director broke my heart by suggesting that, while the "chauffeur's daughter" was in Paris, she actually *buy* a Paris suit. I had to console myself with the dress, whose boat neckline was tied on each shoulder — widely known and copied as "the *Sabrina* neckline."

Audrey and I went shopping in San Francisco; she wanted me as confrere and audience. Shopping is her idea of fun, and no wonder — no matter what she tries on (size eight or nine), she looks simply delicious.

"And now let's celebrate," she'd say when we were exhausted, and that meant heading for the nearest confectionery to devour two of the biggest, fattest, most chocolate French pastries. (When she lived in Holland during the war, food was scarce and she developed a passion for chocolate.)

This girl is one person off stage and on. The charm that made her a star is the same charm she uses when buying a loaf of bread: it's her own personality. And coupled with this charm and magnetism is the mind of a diplomat. If she could run for president, she'd make it. She knows art, music, clothes; she speaks four languages fluently, is shrewd, intelligent, and has an international background; but best of all, she has a positive approach.

Luckily, she's not about to run for president, she's too busy with her two roles, as actress and as Mrs. Mel Ferrer. Incidentally, here is a girl who consults her husband on any personal clothes. Where many women dress for men *before* marriage, and for women *after* marriage, Audrey says it wouldn't be fun to wear clothes unless Mel liked them; and she takes home all sketches for him to see. Of course he likes the clean, uncluttered look that is part of Audrey's personality; he likes, too, the exaggerated use she makes of fashion. High fashion is part of her life, part of her consciousness; she imitates no one.

You have favorite pictures; you can't help it. *Roman Holiday* was one because the clothes were good and Audrey was just right in them. *A Place in the Sun* was another.

Elizabeth Taylor was seventeen at the time — one of the prettiest human beings I've ever seen; gay, enthusiastic and excited about clothes — and let's have no mistake about it, it's fun to dress someone who gets excited. Here we had a perfect setup: one of my favorite producer-directors, George Stevens, and a beautiful star with a flawless young figure playing a girl of wealth.

The clothes were widely copied. One evening gown had countless yards of white tulle studded with countless white velvet violets. One of my young friends reported a party she attended at the time of the picture's release; in attendance were *seventeen* "Elizabeth Taylors" decked in white violets. Another popular dress was a young ball gown of black velvet, topped in eyelet embroidery and studded with seed pearls. I'll always remember Elizabeth saying:

"You can make the waist a little smaller."

"I've already *made* it a little smaller."

"You can make it even a little smaller!"

She had a nineteen-inch waist at the time and she was always trying to get us to make the waists *just* a little smaller.

She was a friendly, uninhibited girl with none of the tricks or traits of the usual child actress who knows she's important and finds a way to let *you* know. Elizabeth wasn't a bit actressish, and she still trotted about the set with her schoolteacher. The teacher came with her to fittings too. I suggested that a couple of fittings might count as schooltime, if we spoke in French and Spanish; but the teacher didn't think that quite legal. Halfway through the picture, Elizabeth graduated, and we had a party in the commissary without the teacher and with everything we could think of fattening to eat. Monty Clift was at the party (he and Elizabeth had become close friends), and the cutter, Tommy McAdoo, and Elizabeth's stand-in and her mother. All very gay.

What impressed me at the time was that Elizabeth was afraid of nothing. She was playing a very taxing picture with a very important producer-director; she showed not the slightest strain; she took each day in stride. I found this same attitude several years later when she suddenly replaced Vivien Leigh in *Elephant Walk*. Many things had happened to Elizabeth:

her first marriage had collapsed; she was now married again, had just had her first baby, and was stepping into the shoes of one of the world's top actresses almost on a moment's notice. She was more sophisticated, and more individual than ever in her beauty; she had acquired a great sureness about clothes and fashion; but she still took each day as it came and dis played not the slightest apprehension about anything.

Where Liz Taylor was of prime importance to me was in that first picture, when she introduced me to the teen-age point of view. I'd had fan mail from teen-agers, but they were teen-agers with problems. From Liz I learned about normal teen-age; and its point of view is a law unto itself. It doesn't necessarily follow the dictates of fashion; it follows its own dictates — and I think it should. This is an age of great crea tivity: they're trying to work out a fashion vocabulary for themselves, and it's a group vocabulary to which a girl had better adhere. It's very unwise to isolate a girl and make her "different." Ask any teen-ager! The objective of the teen-age look is to be very casual when you're casual, and very dressed up when you're dressed up — no in between. Day clothes are underplayed (deliberately of course); evening clothes are far more sophisticated and older than a teen-ager should wear. The day clothes could be worn by a five-year-old, the evening clothes by a twenty-five-year-old.

Elizabeth, at seventeen, was my guide on the teen-age point of view. She sold me completely. I figured if all teen-agers had this *joie de vivre*, they could ignore high fashion.

I didn't know Mitzi Gaynor until she'd grown up, but she tells me she was "awful — fat, long hair, and overdone, if you know what I mean." She gives credit to her husband, Jack Bean, for the present Mitzi; and if he helped her achieve it, more power to him; because she's a girl not in the least subdued.

As you know, I hate third persons at fittings; but Jack came along with Mitzi for *Anything Goes, The Birds and the Bees* and *The Joker Is Wild;* and I found him, far from an interloper, an ally. Mitzi is inclined to look at clothes from her own taste, "I like it" or "I don't like it." Jack is more objective, he knows that clothes have to take a part in the picture. He's a great audience, Mitzi's a great ham; I'm mad about them both.

Essentially, Mitzi can't wait to try on each new style. She's full of exuberance and bounce; when we got her into her "red-spangled strait jacket" for *Anything Goes,* turned on the spotlight and flipped open the doors — Mitzi gave us a show. She has a rounded female figure, good bosom, tiny waist, and she can really sell a costume. If you think she puts on a performance for Jack, you should see her when we finally go down to the set. Some actresses go to the set well hidden in a bathrobe. Mitzi says: "Now, we'll make an entrance" — and does. Everyone whistles, applauds and lifts Mitzi up to the crest of the wave. Every Gaynor costume is a success; it can't lose.

June Allyson, on the other hand, came to me with a firm set of inhibitions about what she could and could not wear.

In *Strategic Air Command,* she played the wife of a flyer and the sweaters and skirts she likes were suitable. However, there was one scene calling for an evening gown with a bare top.

Junie just looked at me. "I don't wear dresses like that."

"Why, June?"

"I don't look well in dresses like that." She went into a long dissertation on the shape of her shoulders (which are actually very nice), the shape of her neck (which is just fine).

Finally I said: "June, let me make it with thin straps. Then, if you're desperately unhappy, we'll make a new top."

The dress was of white Swiss organdy embroidered in cherry red. The bodice was low, with little, thin straps. It was the one dress June bought for her own wardrobe from the picture.

What this girl has is a basic fear of clothes in terms of fashion; she doesn't experiment, she doesn't trust it; and for once, against my usual convictions, I agree. She has built up a June Allyson look, and her public likes it, her family likes it, she likes it. Then, I say, I wouldn't change June. Designers are inclined to make people look like models. But essentially, a model is anonymous, she's a living form to show off clothes. A *person* wears clothes to express personality.

June is the prototype of the girlish American. It's an attractive look, a healthy look, sometimes slightly quaint, and it is June. She's very small, a size five or seven; she can wear clothes well; but she's found her spots and she's not about to change them. I say, more power to *her.*

Ditto Kay Thompson. Here is a woman with such a definite personality she's almost a caricature of herself. She has caricatured her height, her slimness, her brittleness. Many tall, slim women say, "What can I *do* with myself?" Kay shows them, with every gesture.

In *Funny Face* she had a code: a two-piece costume with a short, short skirt and a long, long jacket, a tiny sailor collar at the top. She wore this from tweeds to chiffon. It became a long skirt for evening wear. The point of her uniform was that here was the editor who told every woman what to wear — "Everybody must wear pink!" — but for herself, "I wouldn't be caught dead in it." She announces that every woman must wear different clothes for different moods, and then proceeds to wear her two-piece suit.

Kay, personally, is like a firecracker; she gives vitality to everything she puts on; for fun she assumes the voice of her precocious Eloise, the funny, squeaky voice of a little girl "shot with arsenic." Including Eloise, Kay is completely Kay. This is what each of us is trying for — to be completely one's self.

No one has achieved this better than Miss Katharine Hepburn. She knows how clothes will work for her; she doesn't change with every change of fashion, but she looks fashionable, and you wouldn't dare to say she isn't well dressed. She is. She's developed a technique for being herself and she never makes the mistake of trying to be anyone else.

Miss Hepburn wears high necklines, waists low in back, slightly longer skirts with fullness at the bottom, not the top. She likes gray, pale lemon-yellow, white, and beige, and her basic garment is the shirt. The collar-and-cuff look frames her face. For evening, she wears strapless or sleeveless dresses in rich fabrics, simply made, and always she appears distinguished, smart, utterly Hepburn.

We had a mutual friend, Constance Collier, so I'd heard a good deal about Miss Hepburn, how definite she was, and met her with some trepidation. But *The Rainmaker* was a stimulating experience. "This is the way I usually like clothes made; it'll save us time . . ." said Miss Hepburn, and we proceeded from there. She knows all the tricks; if she wishes to look gauche, the length of the sleeve can show it; the skirt too long achieves an awkward look; so does the belt too wide or too narrow. In the picture, she couldn't have looked less attractive. She played a character brought up with men, in a rural world. In the farm clothes she was enchanting. When she wanted love, and changed herself (her father advised ruffles, flowers and frills), she looked horrible. Very few actresses have the courage to make themselves unattractive; but Miss Hepburn is interested only in the picture. She would use a bit of lace, a red bow, a pinafore, and achieve effect.

I couldn't keep off the set when she was working. The way she walks, talks, the way she moves, crackles with energy. She even puts on shoes like a dynamo. Hers is a driving interest in people, in everything. When she found out I was going to Europe, she started sending me little notes. I was to go *here;* she'd send a list of shops — where I was to go to buy what, what I was to do, what I was to see. It tickled me, because often actresses come to me to ask where they should go. Miss Hepburn *told me.*

So did Eva Marie Saint, but in another way. This delicate-looking blonde arrived in full skirt, sweater and flat shoes, without make-up, a representative of the new school of actresses who do not wish to look like actresses, the Actors' Lab. They all dress the same way, as if by formula. I had seen her in *Waterfront* and on television in *Our Town;* I knew Eva Marie was an actress and a fine one. What Eva Marie told me, very pleasantly but surely, was she did not wish to acquire the "Hollywood look."

The picture was *That Certain Feeling,* a comedy with Bob Hope. It called for very *clothes* clothes. I did not show sketches to her, I was too bright for that. I sat down with her and analyzed the character.

"This is a girl, very New York, very elegant, very feminine," I said. "Two men are in love with her; she is moving in a high-fashion world. It's a part where clothes actually help the story."

It was the right approach. Eva Marie became, at once, a fellow intern. We *took her lining* — the first step in any diagnosis. Off came the full skirt, the sweater, etc., and Eva Marie slipped into a muslin strait jacket that shows all. She has, I discovered, a perfectly good figure. As a matter of fact, eventually she admitted she'd once modeled in New York. But clothes are not her interest. We went into long discussions of the character, what clothes could do to help her change her personality, adapt to the high-comedy tone of the film. There is always the chance that dressing an actress in something she doesn't like can hinder her, at least subconsciously. If she feels unhappy . . . The purpose of our long confabs was to find what would help her, what would hinder her.

The only thing she balked at was jewelry. She wore small pearl earrings and a string of small pearls; costume jewelry she doesn't like and there was no reason she must wear it. The clothes were pretty sensational — very chic, very smart; with the black velvet evening gown we had a velvet stole lined in ermine. Eva Marie fitted and said nothing. I think she was surprised to see what a very different person she could become — and she can, she's versatile. She can be pretty, elegant or drab; speaking clinically, she is a type who can be changed into a number of women. But she said nothing. At the end of the picture she went away; so did I.

When I returned, one of my first phone calls was from Eva Marie Saint. She had seen the picture and wanted me to know how amazing, how really sensational, the clothes had looked! Eva Marie'd never thought of herself as glamorous. I'm not sure she has yet.

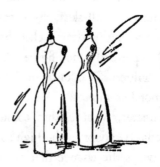

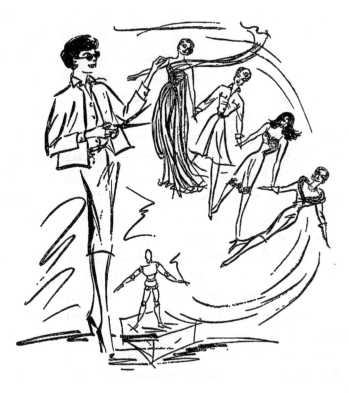

10

Glamorous Guinea Pigs (continued)

I was to meet Rita Hayworth in the very plush offices of Hecht-Hill-Lancaster, than which there are no plushier: one whole wall a cage, filled with exotic-colored birds. It was the emergency call for *Separate Tables*. I'd been alerted the night before at six, read the script at home, I'd rerun Rita Hayworth's last picture that morning; and now, at noon, here I was. I'd never met Miss Hayworth, but I regarded her as a big star; I'd seen press photos of her from all over the world in some of the most wonderful clothes imaginable. One of the most publicized women in the world . . . The love goddess . . . I wore my best Balenciaga suit, uncomfortably high-heeled pumps, handmade suède gloves, a hat you would certainly call smart. And two seconds later, in came Miss Hayworth in blue jeans, tennis shoes and a sweatshirt. She wears no make-up. Her hair was long and loose. She walks quietly, sits quietly; she is one of the shyest people I've ever met.

It was the first in a series of surprises.

Director Delbert Mann discussed the glamorous woman of the play, who is trying to recapture her former husband. She is not a desperate woman, she is a woman trying to be as seductive as possible. I waited for Miss Hayworth to give me the usual pitch. First meetings are usually neat bits of fencing, because nine out of ten actresses come to you with preconceived ideas of what they can wear and what they want. Instead of saying so, they tell you how glad they are you're doing their clothes and that they're leaving *everything* in your hands. Or they tell you how glad they are, and mention casually, "I've always gotten my things at Balmain," or "You know Mainbocher does all my things." In either case, the first meeting means little. At the second meeting, when you show sketches, the actress's true personality begins to show; she tells you *exactly* what she likes or doesn't like, the kind of wardrobe she wants — in short, what she should have said in the first place. (Sometimes, for the second appointment, the actress brings mother, sister, and/or best friend, and asks them what they think. Usual answer, "Well, *I don't know.* . . .")

Miss Hayworth gave me no pitch.

Our second meeting was at her house. She lives near me and suggested I stop by the next day on my way to work. By this time I had some sketches and I was on guard. Now I'd hear exactly what the score was. I think I expected her to be "at home" in a negligee, probably by Elizabeth Arden. Inviting me over could easily be a preamble to showing me a lot of clothes other designers had made for her.

She opened the door looking gay, relaxed and easy — in a pair of golf shorts easily two sizes too large.

"Imagine me talking to a designer in these. I haven't had time to have them made smaller!"

And we looked at sketches. I'd seen the play in New York; so had she, and I thought she'd be interested in how we were interpreting the clothes for the screen. The black dress for the big love scene, for example . . . On Broadway it was of satin with a low V neck. For Rita, I'd suggested a black French wool, embroidered in the smallest black jewels and not such an uncovered dress — certainly not a V neck; she has a pointed face and broad shoulders. The embroidery had a reason, for the love scene on the dark terrace, you could catch body motion by the reflection of light on the tiny gems.

What kind of neckline would Miss Hayworth prefer: square? oval? round?

"I like all of them," she said simply.

I showed her the traveling suit of caramel sheer wool, and waited for reactions. No reactions . . . The more you know about what an actress likes, the easier it is to please her and suit her. You don't want to forcibly superimpose your taste. Rita's only contribution was in the matter of color. She loves warm, tawny color. I decided at once to do everything in tones of her hair and eyes: topaz, sherry, caramel. Although they photograph gray, she'd feel happy in them.

Even in the baggy golf pants, you could see she has an excellent figure — the lean-hipped model look. I knew she'd been dressed by the great designers of the world; I expected her to talk clothes. She did not. She was unworried, disinterested, I thought, until the day she was to arrive for her first fitting. She phoned to say, "I'll be a little late, but it's important, I'm having my hair cut."

Now, what I dislike most in life is the actress who comes to fittings in pincurls (she's going to a party tonight) and who tries on a lovely dress looking like Aunt Jemima. I'd more or less expected Rita in tennis shoes, pincurls and a bandana. She arrived in high heels, hair perfectly dressed, as she'd wear it in the picture!

I'd expected complete disinterest, and certainly her manner had been one of detachment — until she put on the first gown. The minute she was in the fitting, it was like a fire horse hearing the three-alarm. She came to life. She was alert. Nothing interferes with her fitting: no retinue, no agents, no phone calls, no distractions of any kind, and Rita herself says little. Hers were the quietest fittings we've ever had, and, accustomed as we are to exuberant actresses, we weren't really sure she *liked* the clothes. I wasn't sure until the picture was over and Rita went on her wedding trip. The picture of Mr. and Mrs. Jim Hill that broke in the press across country showed Rita in the caramel suit of French wool she'd fitted without comment.

This was a rare time of quiet in the Clinic. Often, when a top star arrives, it's as if a bugle were blowing: royalty. Hal Wallis himself escorted Italian star Anna Magnani — and her interpreter. This was Magnani's first picture in America and it was a big moment, the star talking rapidy in Italian, the rest of us talking English. An explosive moment! Her eyes blazed, her gestures were eloquent, she shook her hair dramatically (she was wearing it in the Magnani manner, and, in the Magnani manner, black slacks and sweater). She shook hands warmly; but if this was a moment of great pleasure, the interpreter failed to convey the message. Hal Wallis introduced us, and left — the coward.

"Tell Miss Magnani how happy I am to work with her. I wish she'd tell me how she sees the character in *The Rose Tattoo*. I know how important clothes are to her in her work."

The interpreter translated this to Italian.

"You have seen my pictures?" asked Magnani.

"Everything you've done," I said quickly. She understood that *without* the interpreter.

"*Bene,*" she said.

We talked back and forth to the interpreter about the blouse and skirt she'd wear in the first scene, before her husband's death. She is a happy woman, she's in love, she goes to the store, it's a normal woman living normally.

"Once the husband dies," I said, "I feel the woman has no interest whatsoever in how she looks."

The interpreter waded back and forth between us. It was pretty heavy going. We got to the scene where she'd wear a slip. Before the interpreter could say a word, Magnani broke in.

"But the slip must not fit well," she said, her black eyes dangerous.

I began to feel an undercurrent. Miss Magnani obviously understood more English than she pretended. Every time I mentioned the word "slip" I felt sparks in the air.

"Material for this slip must not be good," she said.

Ah, she evidently felt that *I* felt all lingerie had to be of handmade silk.

"Disheveled, careless, the slip," she said. "*Décolleté,*" she said. And the way she said it you knew she meant *décolleté.* Her French was beautiful. I switched to French. Los Angeles accent or no, I wasn't getting anywhere in English.

"The clothes should show the disintegration of the woman —from a healthy, lusty woman to a slovenly, dispirited one. *N'est-ce pas?*"

I was doing better.

"At the end, when she is beginning to become more normal, we can get a little glamorous," I said. It was a fatal mistake.

"Never! Tell her — never glamorous!" cried Magnani to the interpreter.

I tried to explain that I was using the word loosely; I meant merely "up from slattern." I went back to the first blouse. "I think a print blouse," I said.

"You have some *old* print blouses?" Magnani asked.

We had; we brought some from Wardrobe and she tried them.

"Let's use these, and make them over," she said, "so the material is not new."

Incidentally, when Magnani undressed, we were amazed. Under the black slacks and sweater was the most exquisite of black French foundations. That night I had a second surprise. The studio had called the press in, to meet the star at a cocktail party. I don't know how I expected her to look; but when I arrived, I was greeted by a handsome, elegant woman in an elegant black silk dress, hair beautifully coiffed, and bearing no resemblance to the woman I'd met earlier in the day. Magnani!

It wasn't until several weeks later that I realized this great actress had been terrified of me, terrified because she was afraid I'd try making her into a Hollywood glamour girl. When she saw the rags I made for her, she began to soften, brighten and blaze. I'll never forget the day we finally became friends. She'd come in to fit the slip, the one costume that had worried her the most, the thing she was afraid would look like French lingerie. It didn't. It was the most dreadful old thing. We'd made it of material from an old slip and constructed it as it might be done in a small Italian town, a bit on the bias at the waist and practically no sewing — no seams, no darts, no fit. Anna took off her own sheer French slip and dragged on this horror. It hung like the original sack.

"*Molte bene!*" she exclaimed to herself in the mirror. "*Molte bene.*"

I laughed. "It hasn't been easy, has it?"

"Not hard," she said. "I worried *before* I met you, Edith. I worried over all the technical people, that they might try to make me over — pluck my eyebrows, you know? I am Magnani! I don't want to be made over." She shook her hair for emphasis.

And again, no designer in her right mind would ever try to change her. She is herself, and she can transform that self completely by the way she wears her hair. She is a robust woman full of gusto, a dramatic actress to the bone; and everyone reflects her. If she is happy, everybody working with her is happy; if she has a headache, she's dying; if something goes wrong, it's a disaster. She's excitable, communicable, emotional — a human Vesuvius; nothing is tranquil, nothing sloughed off, and being around her is exciting. I have seen her explode in her dressing room, tear off the old coat she wore in *Wild Is the Wind*, throw it on the floor and weep with rage. For one awful moment, I thought she was annoyed with the clothes. She wasn't. She was upset over some facet of acting in the scene just shot. But for the most part, she loved the picture and was very gay.

In the beginning of *Wild Is the Wind*, she came bursting in, loaded with good spirits, an armful of magazines with pictures of cowgirls, blue jeans, divided skirts, Stetson hats, and boots she'd had made for herself in Italy. She understood that this was a picture of the Golden West. It was up to me to get the news through to her that this was not a picture about cowboys, but a picture about sheepherders.

She understood English well by now.

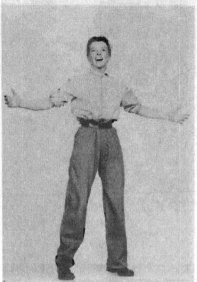

Katharine Hepburn has developed a technique for being herself and nobody else.

(*In* The Rainmaker)

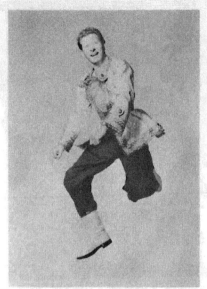

Danny Kaye, who loves to clown, can put a hot water bottle on his head and make it a costume.

(*In* Knock on Wood)

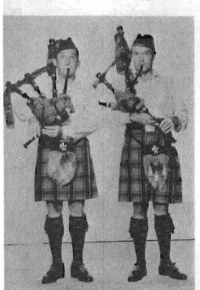

Bing Crosby is the world's fastest fitter. Bob Hope runs the interference.

(*In* The Road to Bali)

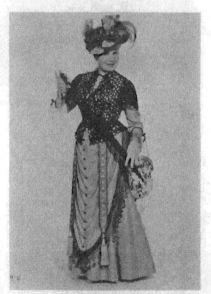

The chic Shirley Booth is a stunning woman. You should see her in the high fashion she wears.

(*In* The Matchmaker)

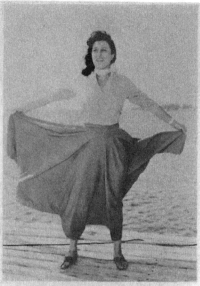

Anna Magnani was afraid I'd try making her over into a Hollywood glamour girl.

(*In* THE ROSE TATTOO)

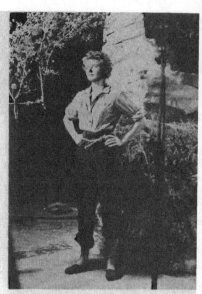

Simplification is the best medicine for making a beautiful woman like Ingrid Bergman more beautiful.

(*In* FOR WHOM THE BELL TOLLS)

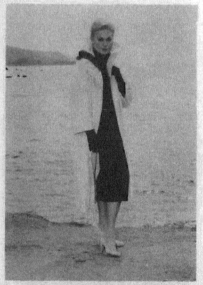

Kim Novak is a lovely female animal with the walk and the figure that make an evening gown look seductive.

(*In* VERTIGO)

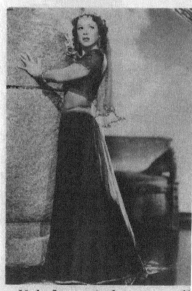

Hedy Lamarr is the most unself conscious siren ever born. She's as relaxed as a Persian cat.

(*In* SAMSON AND DELILAH)

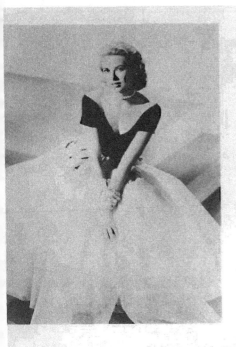

Grace Kelly. It has never seemed strange to me that this girl with her warmth, her poise and her belief in fairy tales should come to live one. (*In* REAR WINDOW)

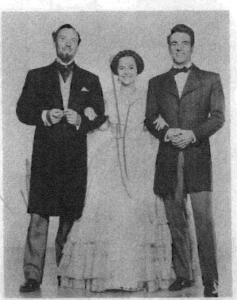

won my first Oscar with *The Heiress*. The problem was to make Olivia de Havilland unattractive.
With Miss de Havilland are Sir Ralph Richardson and Montgomery Clift)

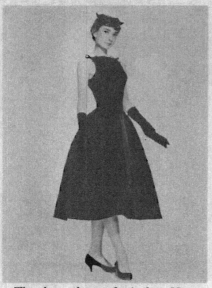

The charm that made Audrey Hepburn a star is the same charm she uses when buying a loaf of bread.
(*In* SABRINA)

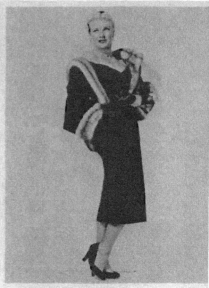

Ginger Rogers is apple-pie American. She puts on a costume like a girl getting ready for a high-school prom.
(*In* FOREVER FEMALE)

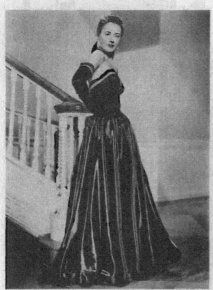

Barbara Stanwyck is extraordinarily honest, brutally frank, and absolutely loyal.
(*In* THE BRIDE WORE BOOTS)

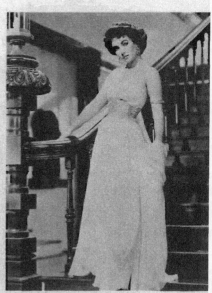

Elizabeth Taylor at seventeen was my guide on the teen-age point of view.
(*In* ELEPHANT WALK)

"There's a fine sartorial difference between a sheepman and a cowman," I said.

Magnani laughed heartily. Everyone laughed with her. And I turned her loose in Wardrobe to try on endless pants, boots, coats and dresses.

The one dress to be made was for the party scene, when her husband has given her money and she's bought a dress. We did a middle-class, American-looking party dress. It was a *disaster.* "It is not possible," she said. "I will bring in one of my own dresses; it is just right."

She designs her own clothes, incidentally; and simple and smart, even stark, they are. The one she brought in was a sheath with a loose back panel that hung from the shoulders. It was sleeveless, high-necked, very dramatic, made of heavy, black Italian silk. "This is my original design," she said. "Never let any other actress have it. You, personally, may copy it." We made it for her in black linen, embroidered with hot pink carnations. We had regained the Magnani look.

A *look* is every woman's aim. For Jane Russell, it's a sexy look, so that even when I had her for a western, *Son of Pale-face,* with nothing but cowgirl outfits, they had to be Jane Russell clothes. Where the average western costume looks as if you were really going out to rope cattle, Jane's looks as though she couldn't possibly rope anything but men. I used glove suède for Jane's cowgirl clothes, because glove suède clings — and that's what it did, all over.

For Pearl Bailey, it's a bouncy, gay, sexy look, and even

when she plays a maid, as she did in *That Certain Feeling*, the maid's costume was fitted like a ball gown.

For Eartha Kitt, it's a sexy pussycat look. She has a true feline quality and the fringe on her costumes never quite lies down.

For Doris Day, it's a clean-cut, crisp, typically American look. When Doris first arrived for *The Man Who Knew Too Much*, she said: I'm not going to tell you what I like or what I don't like; I'm in your hands, Edith — dress me."

She was absolutely safe. Doris is such a definite type, she looks so well in what she wears, you couldn't possibly change her. I'd hate to have to dress her as Scarlet O'Hara. I think the secret of her smartness is that she's found the clothes in which she feels comfortable. If the effect today is casual, its achievement was not. I discovered that when I reran her old pictures. Look at those early films and you see a grown-up Meglin Kiddie, replete with buttons, bows, ruffles and curls, who bears no resemblance to today's Doris. I was amazed. Then I ran *Julie*, her first independent production, and an abrupt departure from what had gone before. Here Doris emerged with clipped hair, she wore her own clothes, and she was *right*. I dressed her exactly as she dresses in *The Man Who Knew Too Much*. For *Teacher's Pet*, as a journalism teacher, she wore suits. Here we had no trouble, Doris loves suits. Trouble appeared in the shape of the one dress for the nightclub sequence. My point of view was that when the journalism instructress went out she would dress more softly, less casually, offering contrast to what she usually wore.

We made a dozen sketches, and finally compromised on a cocktail dress, but a plain one.

Doris worried over that dress. She's a chronic worrier — but only about clothes. Otherwise, she's full of vitality and full of zip, and very much a little girl. We went shopping one day. She bought all kinds of things, things she needed and shoes and hats she didn't need at all, but they were so pretty. In each store she has salespeople who know her, and there is the friendliest, warmest relationship between Doris and these people. She's one actress who is spontaneous and unaffected, and, as she says, "gets a bang" out of little things.

"I'm hungry," Doris said, in the middle of shopping, and steered me to Biff's lunch counter. Most actresses would have selected the Derby, or Romanoff's, or Frascati's, and they'd nibble on lettuce leaves. Doris ordered two cheeseburgers with everything on them, and the biggest malted milks I've ever seen. She enjoyed this as if it were her last chance at food for the week. Two hours later, in her dressing room, I found her eating graham crackers piled with peanut butter.

"This is one of the dreamiest things in the world," she said. "Let me make you one!" As someone else might say, "Let me show you my latest Picasso!"

Doris is a blow to a designer, because in sweater, skirt and no make-up she looks as well as when you've worked on her, doing your best. Glamour adds nothing; it detracts from her.

Many of today's young stars have good figures; they're pretty, but they're in a new tradition — they don't look like stars, off screen. Janet Leigh could be the young clubwoman; Vera Miles, Ann Blyth, Hope Lange, Joanne Woodward, Kathy Grant, Diana Lynn, Debbie Reynolds, Jean Simmons, Natalie Wood could be pictured easily on the society page rather than the movie page. And then there are the individualists, like Carolyn Jones and Shirley MacLaine. Shirley fits into no mold or pigeonhole. She's the most completely uninhibited, completely honest person I've ever met.

"Edith, you may think this is elegant," she'll say; "I think it's awful."

"Why?"

"I look like everybody else!"

I make some change — skirt length, sleeve length or belt, so that Shirley feels like Shirley. A designer should not force her taste, and the individual with strength to be the individual has the assurance that is one of clothes' prime objectives. Shirley has it.

I may say, "Shirley, how are you going to wear your hair to the Academy Awards?"

"Like this," she'll say — "upswept haystack."

I don't always agree, but who asks me? Not Shirley. Not Carolyn.

Carolyn Jones has manufactured a personality for herself, and it's paid off. She'd been around here for some time, a naturally pretty blond stock girl who was getting nowhere. Then she dyed her hair dark, developed bangs, a big, blue-eyed stare, a different kind of talk, a different kind of walk, everything. Now her approach is very positive and electric;

on screen she can wear extreme clothes: the wool and cellophane dress that looked like a wet snake in *King Creole*, the slinky black number in *Showdown Hill*. Carolyn's clothes on screen are clothes designed as male bait, and when she shows them, she *shows* them: "Isn't this just the jazziest, Mr. Wallis?" wriggling along in pale-green jersey that is strictly an eyecatcher.

Carolyn and Shirley are little laws unto themselves; but most young actresses want help, need help, and, fashionwise, they're quick-change artists, they learn faster than their more established sisters.

Dolores Hart arrived here one year ago, an eighteen-year-old student from Marymount College in a blouse, a skirt and a pony tail; I nicknamed her "Junior." What has happened to Dolores in one year is unbelievable. Her first picture was *Loving You* with Elvis Presley. She played a fresh-faced girl, very pretty. Then she played with Anna Magnani in *Wild is the Wind*, then nothing much happened except that her name kept appearing on fan-magazine polls and she made *King Creole* with Presley. Her first real break was on Broadway in *The Pleasure of His Company*. Day after the opening, unknown Dolores was the rave of New York. Next big break, opposite Montgomery Clift in *Lonelyhearts*.

Dolores just phoned.

"This is 'Junior,'" she said. "I'm going East for personal appearances. Should I look like myself or like an actress?"

"Like an actress who looks like herself," I said, "Come on up."

She was leaving so quickly she had no time to buy clothes, or to have all her own in readiness; we had to lend her some things from Wardrobe. Not screen clothes, and not glamorous clothes: slim skirts, jackets, blouses — interchangeable. We used only three colors: black, beige and white, and I gave her a chart of what shoes, bags, etc. to wear with each combination, so when she's in a hurry she won't have to think.

Like everyone else on the lot, I wanted this girl to make it. She's as friendly and trusting as a kitten; she's not *on* like many actresses, she's ambitious, but she has such a quick curiosity about life that acting isn't the end and all. The first day she came to the Clinic, we talked about animals. Like myself, Dolores loves anything that crawls, jumps, flies or walks on four legs. I mentioned the horned toads I'd played with when I was a little girl. The next day I received a present — a horned toad in a little cage. I've been given some handsome gifts in my time, but never a horned toad; and I couldn't have been more pleased. The toad is at present residing at Rex Ellsworth's ranch, close enough to Khaled, the famous stallion, to enjoy the same flies.

The qualities so beguiling about the girl are her eagerness, her healthy, young look, and the absence of star complex. In a year she changed from a schoolgirl to a graceful young woman, and clothes helped give her some of this new assurance. Before Dolores, as before all young actresses, I hold up the image of my very favorite guinea pig — Grace Kelly. Grace has a look I love. There is no pretense in her make-up or her clothes; she never dressed to attract attention; she never dressed like an actress; she dressed like Grace Kelly, and she was Grace Kelly — which didn't keep her from becoming varied characters on screen.

In two of the four pictures Grace Kelly and I worked in together, I was able to translate her from the high-fashion model of *Rear Window* to the drab, dull housewife of *Country Girl*. For the drab, we tried all kinds of sweaters and house-dresses as she certainly didn't want to look like a caricature of "Little Eva." The dress had to look as if she'd worn it a long time, as if she'd lost a great deal of weight, and so on. We found, finally, a shapeless wraparound housedress and a sweater that had been in stock for years; we put them through a washing machine, "aged" them, and called Bill Holden in for a masculine reaction. He assured us Grace looked not in the least Grace. She felt very definitely that without this physical change to help her, it would have been most difficult to play the part.

Usually, she played the charming, well-bred cultured person she is, a girl who has traveled all her life, who has known money all her life, and is used to good clothes. Hitchcock had told me I'd have a field day, that the girl had the model look, but I'd seen her only in *High Noon* and I wasn't prepared.

She came up the stairs briskly that first day, looking like a girl just out of Bryn Mawr — the whitest of white gloves, the whitest of blouses, the gray tailored suit, the tailored hat, the most immaculate scrubbed look! We're used to a certain amount of careless dressing in Hollywood; nothing about

Grace was careless. Even better than the clothes was the quiet, shy, interested manner; she becomes articulate and gay as she gets to know you, and hers is a childlike ability to be pleased. In the pale, frothy negligee of *Rear Window,* she positively giggled at her image in the mirrors.

"Why, I look like a peach parfait," she said. "Call the girls in; let them see!" We were both delighted with the suit of Celadon-green raw silk with its straight box jacket, its wide neckline and tight hip. The suit was the one Hitchcock had first seen in his mind's eye, colorwise; and it caused a furore fashionwise.

What Grace has is an elegance all her own; the white gloves are a trade mark, so is the smooth hair. She looks that way even after sleeping all night on a plane. I met her at the airport when she arrived in France for *To Catch a Thief.* I'd gone over earlier to do clothes for the French members of the cast; then we were on location on the Riviera for six weeks. But first we had a few days in Paris. We bought bags and shoes (typically French) to go with her clothes in the picture; we hunted for a French bathing suit (after seeing the bikinis, we settled for an American suit). I got to *know* Grace in Paris. We went to the tennis matches (anyone who thinks her reserved has never gone with her to watch tennis); we went shopping at Hermés, where she bought presents for every member of her family — gloves. We went to the theater; we ate beautiful food and drank beautiful wine.

Often, the Hitchcocks were with us; Alfred Hitchcock is a great gourmet.

Later, back in America, Grace had a party for Alfred and Alma Hitchcock and served all the delicacies he'd liked best. "This is what you ate at the Plaza Athenée! And this is what you ate at . . ." Grace never was THE ACTRESS; she liked acting, and did it well, but it was just another experience; she was a girl who believed in life. She loved beauty, loved prettiness, and wasn't afraid to tell you so. She was mad about children and carried pictures of her sister's and her brothers' children. She was close to her family, and when her mother, aunt and sisters came to the coast, she brought them to all fittings. You know my well-founded dread of relatives; but the Kelly clan came to observe and appreciate, the way they'd go to the theater. I actually surprised myself and *asked* Grace to bring them.

When she was on location, she'd send little notes back. The day before she left here to be married, we had lunch together at Paramount, and she showed me pictures of her prince. You should have seen the look on her face when people dropped by the table to ask when she was coming back. "Coming back? I'm going to get married," she said, like any other girl in love. Show business was part of the past, like school and college. I receive notes from her now, pictures of the children, the other day an enchanting book of old costumes from Switzerland. Before that, a handkerchief from Paris. And I've sent her children their first little white gloves. She keeps her same girlish delight and enthusiasm, the same rose-colored glasses she was born wearing.

Reporters besieged me at the time of the wedding, wanting

anecdotes about the new Princess of Monaco. "You must know some anecdotes."

"Grace doesn't allow anecdotes to happen to her," I told them. And she doesn't. She doesn't enjoy public notice. When she was living at the Bel Air Hotel, she loved to bring her sister and have picnics out in our garden, loved to go swimming there completely alone. She could never see that being a professional person entailed the forfeit of privacy.

Of the clothes I made Grace, what I liked best was the ice-blue satin dress for the opening of *Country Girl*. She wired me from Philadelphia that time asking for a dress; I made it and sent it. Later she wore it when she won her Academy Award. I loved, too, the golden princess dress from *To Catch a Thief*.

It never has seemed strange to me that this girl, with her warmth, her poise and her belief in fairy tales, should come to live one. As I tell the young hopefuls dressing in her image: "You too can become a princess."

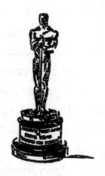

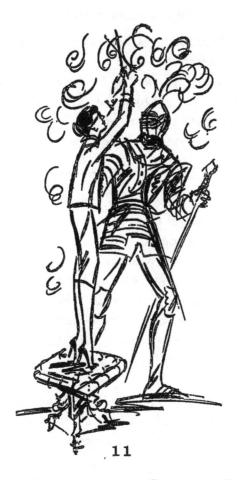

11

The Masculine Point of View

To LOOK LOVELY, a woman will suffer. She'll wear a waist cincher that squeezes her, boned bras that dig her, heels that tilt her to the sensitive balls of her feet, earrings that pinch, skirts too tight for walking, belts too tight for breathing. No man will do it. Only one thing matters to the gentlemen who've wandered into my Clinic (some of them at the point of a gun) — COMFORT.

I learned that early from Bing Crosby when we were working on *Holiday Inn*; and from that day to this, Bing has held his record as WORLD'S FASTEST FITTER. He doesn't like dress-up, he'd never dream of it unless the script so demanded; his famous first words are always, "Why don't we wear a sport coat?"

Let me explain that my job includes complete costume supervision of each picture: man, woman, child and camel. But, unless the picture is a period piece or a comedy, actors usually wear their own wardrobe. So when Bing begs for a sport coat in my fitting room, it's because he's trapped on *The Road to Morocco* or worse, in *White Christmas*, when he and Danny Kaye had to improvise a "sister" act! Bing took one look at the scarves and fans, the jeweled butterfly I was about to stick in his hair, and set his ears back.

"You kidding?"

Luckily, Danny, who loves to clown — who can put a hot-water bottle on his head and make a costume — immediately seized scarf and fan and began a kicking routine. With him to help and while Bing waggled a golf club (his favorite prop while fitting), we got him rigged up as something that hilariously suggested a chorus girl.

What makes Bing the world's fastest fitter is that he's strictly a fugitive from masquerade. The best way to trap him is with the co-operation of a Danny Kaye or a Bob Hope. Most of his costumes have been for pictures Bing and Bob made together, and Bob runs the interference. For him it's a pleasure. He adores costume pictures in which he can be sheik, sultan or Spanish dancer, and he lives it up. He can't put on anything without reacting to it — smirking at the dragon up the back of his Chinese pajamas, rolling his eyes under a turban. The more he reacts, the funnier it gets; and Bing can't resist, like a patient under laughing gas. The contagion spreads throughout the Clinic; their fittings are as funny as the finished picture.

Bob not only reacts to his own clothes, he reacts madly to whatever his leading lady wears. I've seen him break them up, from Dorothy Lamour to Eva Marie Saint. When Hedy Lamarr appeared for *My Favorite Spy* in a glittering gown so tight she couldn't walk she had to slither, and with one shoulder bared, Bob took a look and stage-whispered: "Who's going to look at me in this scene?"

I didn't realize how aware Bing was of women's clothes, however, until he brought me my first toreador shirts from Spain. This was long before I'd been to Spain or succumbed to the charm of Spanish fashion. Just before he'd left for Europe, he'd found me very upset one day. A columnist had named the ten *worst* dressed women in Hollywood, and among them, me. The columnist was objecting to my "uniform": the tailored suits and tailored shirts I've worn purposely. Bing told me to pay no attention to the columnist and quoted a few choice tidbits the same writer had tossed at him. But when he returned from his trip, he brought me these beautiful toreador shirts, he'd had them made for me of ruffled white broadcloth. "You just wear these with your suits," he said.

Another man extremely observant of what women wear is Cary Grant, and I use him frequently as medical consultant. Cary has lived everywhere; he has international background; his taste is impeccable. (I consider him not only the most beautiful but the most beautifully dressed man in the world.) When we were making *Houseboat*, I talked to him about clothes for Martha Hyer who was supposed to live near Washington, D.C., a member of the country club set. I've been all over the world but I never have been to a country club dance with the summer set near Washington. Cary, I knew, had lived there. So I checked him to see if summer cottons would be correct for the dance. They would be, he assured me, and men would not wear dinner clothes, the whole thing is most informal.

You can trust Cary Grant. His is a discerning eye, a meticulous sense of detail. When we were making *To Catch a Thief*, he came up to the Clinic and planned a color scheme for his wardrobe throughout the picture. He found what Grace Kelly was wearing in each scene, then selected clothes to complement hers. "She's wearing a pale blue bathing suit for the beach scene? Good, I'll wear plaid shorts. She's wearing a gray dress? How would it be if I wear a dark jacket and gray slacks?" That he admired the clothes I'd done for Grace was my best assurance and insurance.

Does it surprise you that men are authoritative on the subject of women's clothes? They not only are, they've taught me a great deal by showing me their point of view. Carolyn Jones walks on the set of *A Hole in Your Head* and Frank Sinatra's face lights up, he gives me a big wink and sighs, "That's a *gasser!*" Clothes, Sinatra language, are either gassers or nothing, just as the femme who wears them is exciting or not; and director Frank Capra wanted Carolyn's wardrobe to be so exciting and Eleanor Parker's so conservative that the audience would respond to these girls without a word of dialogue. Frank responded. Marlon Brando, on the other hand, doesn't notice clothes unless they're wrong. "I never separate a dress from an actress. I'm concerned only with the reality she conveys. If the dress is wrong, reality's lost," he says. Jerry Lewis, the do-it-yourselfer of the industry, who constantly improvises gag costumes, grabbing things out of Wardrobe while you stand helplessly by — this same Jerry, producing his own pictures, keeps an eagle and very serious eye on his leading lady's clothes.

"If you are playing a scene with a girl who is supposed to be sweet, simple and sympathetic, and she looks like a witch in clothes too tight, too low and too siren — no matter how good an actress is, you feel a psychological barrier. You can't think of her as a grown-up Girl Scout," Jerry says. "If this is true in comedy, how much more true in serious drama, and how much more true in *real life*. What a woman wears creates, subconsciously, your idea of what she is. In every scene I'm aware, as an actor, of the impact the actress is making on *me* and at the same time I'm aware, as a producer, of what the audience is going to think." Then Jerry really floored me.

He said, "You know, I've always admired the way you dress, Edith. When you show me sketches you're not competing with either the sketches or with the actress. It's damned smart." I had no idea this Jerry was so observant.

Yul Brynner and I talk endlessly on the psychology of clothes; over lunch in the commissary, day after day, when he's here, we match verbal swords. Yul thinks most clothes are too "self-conscious" — they overpower the actress; they interfere with audience perception. That's why men are often more effective than women on screen, he says. Men's clothes are simpler, the audience can concentrate on their characterizations. In *The Buccaneer,* for example, he felt that Claire Bloom in her ordinary pirate clothes was far more dramatic than she or Inger Stevens in their jeweled ball gowns. It is something for a designer to think about, for a doctor to put into practice.

Every woman, and certainly every designer, needs the masculine reaction. Most men are, clotheswise, conservative, a trifle old-fashioned; and they embarrass easily. When a man puts his arms around a girl's waist, he doesn't want to feel a corset. If he puts his arm across her shoulders, he doesn't want to confuse her with a football hero. They don't like lampshade tunics, exaggerated peplums, hobbleskirts, trick necklines or gadgets. They dislike clothes cut too low, too short or that are too attention-getting. They like provocative clothes, but they don't want that provocation handed them on a silver platter. They like glamour in fabric or in design but not both. They love women in black. They like suits, but loathe those that look like female versions of their own They object to clothes which are obviously young or obviously sophisticated. In a situation where Clark Gable is torn between two women, his divorced wife (Lilli Palmer) and his secretary (Carroll Baker), producers Bill Perlberg and George Seaton insist we avoid any great contrast in clothes. They don't want Lilli dressed to telegraph the point that she's more urbane or Carroll dressed to proclaim how young and ingenue she is. Why tip their hand storywise? Good clothes have no *age*. Above all, clothes should be comfortable. Men always want women to look as if they were comfortable and at ease.

The six men with whom I've worked who have influenced me most are: Alfred Hitchcock, George Stevens, Hal Wallis, William Wyler, George Cukor and Cecil B. de Mille. These skilled specialists in the art of picture making are clinical to the nth degree, and they've taught me many things. First and foremost: in designing clothes for women there is one thing to keep in mind — MEN!

"The trouble with most designers," says Hal Wallis, "they think only of what women will like. The very dress that may delight women in the audience may appall every man."

Hitchcock thinks in terms of color; every costume is indicated when he sends me the script. For Grace Kelly in *Rear Window* he wanted especially a "pale green suit"; for the fancy dress ball in *To Catch a Thief* he saw her in gold. There is always a story reason behind his thinking, an effort to characterize. He's absolutely definite in his visual approach, and gives you an exciting concept of the importance of color.

When he signed Vera Miles, he asked me to study her. "She's an extraordinarily good actress, but she doesn't dress in a way that gives her the distinction her acting warrants," he said. I saw what he meant. When you walked in a room and saw Vera you thought, "A pretty, pretty girl," not *"Who is she?"*

"She's not outstanding," Hitchcock said, "because she uses too much color. She's swamped by color. I think the reason I was impressed with her to begin with was that I saw her in black and white on television." So we reduced Vera to black and white photography. I did a complete personal wardrobe for her when she was first presented in New York: black, white and gray. Now Vera wouldn't think of wearing any other colors, in black, white and gray she feels right, as I do in black, white or beige. People are forever telling me I should wear red. In red I feel like a lost fire engine. Hitchcock's color sense rubs off!

George Stevens has no preconceived ideas about color. He leaves it to me to go through the script and illustrate it as if it were a book. *A Place in the Sun* or *Shane* is first worked out in terms of illustration before it begins to move around on the set. He wants realism, not prettiness. He was impressed with the beautiful Elizabeth Taylor rich-girl wardrobe for *A Place in the Sun;* but he was crazy about the funny clothes we found for Shelley Winters by going to bargain-basement sales.

Hal Wallis is the toughest. All clothes for his pictures *must* be understated. He doesn't want to be *conscious* of clothes. He wants nothing to interfere with telling the story.

"But Hal, this is smarter," you may say.

"Good; save it for the next fashion show!"

Whether we're conveying the stark realism of a Shirley Booth, the dramatic characterization of a Katharine Hepburn, the clowning mood of a Jerry Lewis comedy, the offbeat tempo of an Elvis Presley picture — story comes first to Hall Wallis. Nothing must clutter the point of view.

When Willie Wyler makes a black-and-white picture, he wants only black-and-white sketches (we usually do all sketches in color). He is completely the realist. Audrey Hepburn in *Roman Holiday* had to look like an everyday girl in the streets of Rome, not like the princess she was. Olivia de Havilland in *The Heiress* had to look as if no human being would marry her except for her money, in an era when almost every dress was beautiful. There can be no fudging, no extra hint of softening. He wants no model sketch either, but a sketch that looks exactly like what he's going to see on screen, with the figure drawn like the figure of the actress. Normally, a designer sketches an elongated, stylized dream of a figure: tall, long-legged, tiny-waisted, slim-hipped — a willowy clotheshorse. Willie wants none of that. If the actress is short and broad, draw her short and broad, and the dress as it will fit. He wants real women walking around in his mind's eye, and on his screen.

So does George Cukor. Most sensitive to clothes, he works closely with a designer, even comes to fittings. Cukor's influence on me dates back to pictures like *Camille* which I admired from an enormous distance. His is the theater point of view and he has a phobia against anything the least hackneyed. "Don't start digging out a flock of cowboy outfits," he told me as we contemplated a western with Sophia Loren. "This is a dramatic picture in a western atmosphere, let's not make it look like a TV serial!" He hates formula, he won't tolerate an actress emerging like a stereotype. By coming to fittings, he keeps an eye on every detail and details count.

De Mille is master of the super production, a perfectionist on the encyclopedic detail demanded by his plunges into history. When you do the headdress for Nefertiri, you'd better be prepared to quote volume and page to verify that this will match the replica found in the Egyptian queen's very tomb.

He never shows enthusiasm. No "Wonderful!" No "Beautiful!" No "Good, Edith!" Once I said to him, "Mr. de Mille, in all these years we've worked together, you've never told me a costume was good. The most you say is, 'That will do.' "

He almost smiled. "If I say it will do, it's good!"

De Mille wants color sketches always; he has a color print made of the sketch and blows it up giant-size, to compare with the finished costume when you finally show it. If the original sketch had seven pearls on the shoulder strap, if the drape revealed the leg to halfway between knee and thigh, be quite certain the finished costume is identical.

For the ending of *Samson and Delilah*, the temple scene, I sketched Hedy Lamarr in peacock blues and greens with a long flowing cape to suggest the bird.

"Why not use real peacock feathers?" asked Mr. de Mille. "Make a whole dress of peacock feathers."

"They're almost impossible to get," I said.

"No peacock feathers?"

"I tried not long ago to get some for a Lamour turban," I said. "But even if we could get the feathers, I think it would be almost impossible to make a dress of them.

My mistake. It was like waving a red flag before a very active bull.

"You used to teach school, didn't you, Edith? Well now, you've heard of a durbar?"

"Isn't that the ceremonial in which the rulers of India receive visitors of state?"

"It is, indeed; and at the durbar ball in 1903 Lady Curzon caused a sensation. On page so and so of such a such a book you will find a picture of Lady Curzon's dress. It was made entirely — of *peacock feathers!* If they could do it then, we can do it now. I'll supply the feathers," he said.

A few days later, a station wagon filled with plumage arrived, M. de Mille at the wheel.

"I have a ranch," he explained. "We raise peacocks. I just spent the week end picking up fallen feathers."

So, I designed and we made a magnificent dress that transformed Hedy into the most exotic of birds. Mr. de Mille was so proud of it he took it home when the picture ended. (I might also add that the picture brought me an Academy Award, toward which the peacock dress probably contributed no little.) From Mr. de Mille you learn the importance of accuracy and absolute authenticity.

Charlton Heston, on the other hand, is constantly trying to coerce me into poetic license. At least, so goes our running gag. It started when he came up to Surgery just before *The Greatest Show on Earth*. He arrived while I was working on a sketch, painting in sequins, and strings of sequins were draped over the drawing board.

"Are those spangles?" he asked.

"Academically, no. Those are sequins, also known as pail-lettes."

"Will I wear them?"

"You will not."

"Why? Is there any reason why I can't wear sequins?"

"Well-uh, yes," I said. I, who hate people who start sentences with Well-uh or But-uh . . . "You aren't playing a trapeze performer."

"Cornel Wilde gets sequins?"

"He's an acrobat."

Each time Charlton came up for his fittings, he'd see glittering trappings for everyone else in the picture.

"Everyone in the circus wears glitter but me?" he'd say.

"Yes. The only man in the circus who doesn't glitter is the man behind the scenes."

He looked quite downcast! Now, I'm sure Charlton Heston wouldn't be caught dead in sequins; but he heckled me constantly, to no avail. He didn't get sequins in *The Ten Commandments* or in *The Buccaneer* or any of his pictures, and he continues to plague me. When my husband and I were visiting in Rome during the filming of *Ben Hur*, we were sitting at lunch with Willie Wyler, Audrey Hepburn and an assortment of international press representatives, when Charlton joined us.

"Where are my sequins?" he said.

"Aren't you wearing them in *Ben Hur*?" I asked sweetly, *Ben Hur* not being our picture and my responsibility nil. I've stood my ground for at least half a dozen pictures with this persuasive man. If someday you see him bound onto the screen shimmering, you'll know I've lost the pleasant battle.

If all this sounds as if I enjoy working with gentlemen patients, I *do*. The most fun we ever have at this Clinic is when Danny Kaye arrives and completely disrupts the place.

"Where're my sketches? Where's food? Why aren't things being done?" he'll yell, bounding up the stairs a good three weeks before sketches are due or himself expected. And there he stands, leaning against the door, a sartorial hodgepodge in duck pants, nature-boy shoes, silly golf hat and magnificent alpaca sweater (he has a handsome collection of sweaters and likes them appreciated).

"This is terrible, no one cares!" he moans while we dissolve in mock sorrow. He loves huge sandwiches, cookies, Cokes; these necessities appear immediately because everyone on the staff loves Danny, he can do no wrong. *And* he's genuinely interested in costume. When we're at the deciding stage, he's dead serious.

It goes like this. Say we're working on costumes for *The*

Five Pennies, the story of Red Nichols. We have the place set up like an art gallery, costume sketches propped up around the room, bolts of tweeds and cashmeres, rich fabrics a man with means would wear. Red Nichols started out poor, but became a successful man, and since the period of the picture is the 20's and 30's, today's clothes won't do. Danny arrives with director, Mel Shevelson, producer Jack Rose, the cameraman, art director, color consultant, etc., and they march around the room studying each sketch and fabric seriously. Shevelson and Rose are more interested in how an actor looks than in how an actress looks. In *Houseboat* they were perfectly willing to stretch a point and have Sophia wear clothes more glamorous than she would have worn applying for a job as housekeeper, because it made her entrance so funny. But in this instance, what Danny wears influences his interpretation and that's important. Danny leads the parade around the room, his hands deep in his pockets, dead pan, dead silence, studying each sketch, each fabric seriously, intently, not a word — not at all the Danny Kaye we know. After he's examined each thing with care, he sits down. We *all* sit down, and wait. Does he like what we've done? Doesn't he? Then suddenly . . .

"Edith," Danny says, "*why* do women wear girdles?"

The place falls apart. That's Danny again. But when we get *that* matter settled, he is ready to discuss seriously what he's going to wear as Red Nichols to show the transition of time, age, locale and financial position. On the screen, the character can't say, "I'm ten years older now and have money!"

You prove it by clothes and attitude. Danny discusses and we decide on each costume for each scene of the picture. There's not a trace of zanyness, it would be in the way. Once we've decided, he explodes.

"Food!" he yells. "Food, food, food!" A few minutes later, beaming happily, he's sitting cross-legged on the floor eating.

It's the change of pace that makes him so funny, and funny is what this man is, in spite of the fact that he is basically a handsome man (who works hard at not being a handsome man). In *The Court Jester*, in tights, black velvet doublet and plumes he could have looked magnificent. Only his acting saved him. In *Me and the Colonel* only his mustache saved him.

Like my other male patients, although he's very concerned about authenticity and characterization, his chief concern is comfort. The nearest he and I ever came to a struggle was when *The Court Jester* called for a suit of armor.

"A nice comfortable suit of armor?" Danny said.

I must have looked dubious. I know some tricks but they don't include comfortable armor.

"Let's drop the picture," Danny said and meant it.

Director-producers Panama and Frank looked at me in despair. It was up to me; and finally, with the help of modern science, I was able to entice Danny into a suit of flexible aluminum. Even so, he hated it.

Just as Tony Perkins hated his tight, narrow-shouldered suit for *The Matchmaker*. He'd try on the jackets with their tight collars, their small-town gawky look; we'd button them up, he'd expand his chest. Pop! Finally, to get Tony before the cameras for this period piece, I had to make his clothes look tight without their actually being too tight.

So far as fashion goes, the men have one word 'for it — COMFORT.

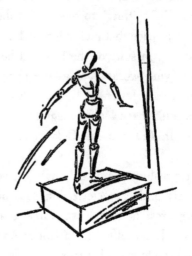

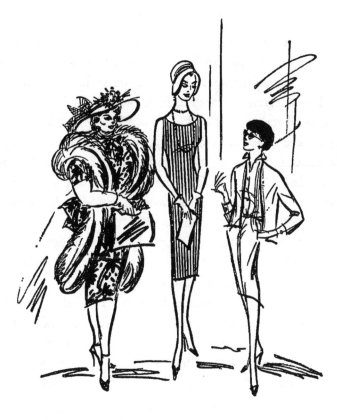

12

Guinea Pigs Who Need Glamour

HOLLYWOOD IS NOT necessarily the greatest fashion center of the world, but motion pictures being the largest means of mass communication, fashions seen on the screen have an enormous effect. From the time I was a trembling intern, never sure of my next operation, fan letters have been coming in: movie fans admired a certain dress, wanted a pattern. I couldn't send a pattern, but I did send little sketches. The minute Dorothy Lamour hit the screen in her first sarong, the fan mail grew. It continued to grow with the Latin American trend started in *The Lady Eve*. *Women's Wear Daily* reproduced adaptations of the guayavera (Mexican shirt), the poncho, the serape styles, and identified them as "Edith Head designs." Other fans wrote in for the pattern of a certain wedding dress; others wrote wanting to know how to look better, more glamorous.

I have always observed people. From that first trip to Europe, I've spent every cent and all my leisure traveling and SEEING how women look everywhere. If Billy Wilder says, "You know those women in Soho . . ." I do know. If producers Carlo Ponti and Marcello Girosi talk of Italian widows in mourning — *The Black Orchid* — I know the kind of women of whom they speak. If Delbert Mann is discussing Rita Hayworth's clothes for a small hotel on the seacoast of England . . . But I also observe people here in America. I visit supermarkets and Sears Roebuck stores, watch women in bargain basements and cafeteria lines, in swank department stores buying clothes, at laundromats and at first nights. I'm getting ideas for the actresses I must transform into character, yes; but also, I'm dying to tap women on the shoulder, nice-looking women, overdressed or dowdy women who should be told, "Mrs. Average American, you could look lovely. Even on a limited budget, you don't have to look middle-aged or negative. Now, what you should wear is this. . . ."

In January 1945 I suddenly, surprisingly, got my chance. Art Linkletter started a new radio program. The audience was composed of everyday women, not chi-chi fashion-conscious women, but homemakers accustomed to doing their own housework and raising their own children; and Linkletter invited a guest expert on each program — Perc Westmore to tell them about make-up; an expert on figure control; a family relations counsellor. Would I come on, discuss clothes, walk through the audience and actually tell women what was wrong with the way they looked?

Would I! I've never been afraid of talking to *any* group of women, any size. As for snap judgments, I've made them daily. This was my chance to turn America into a country of neat and natty women, women with assurance, women who *knew* they looked *right.*

The next think I knew, a microphone was in front of my face, Art Linkletter had me by the arm and we were walking down the aisle through a crowded auditorium. At least Art was walking, he practically carried me. Something about that bit of metal on a cord corrupted all the muscles I'd once built at the YWCA. "This is Edith Head of Paramount, she's trained to help the stars dress beautifully, perhaps she can help you," Art said smoothly. "Just stand and ask your questions. Ah, this lady in the fifteenth row . . ."

She stood up. "Is my dress right?" she said.

I eyed her wildly. Silence on radio is dead air, I had to talk and talk fast, and this woman had on everything but a tiara: flowered dress, flowered hat, fancy shoes, fancy gloves and tons of jewelry. I said:

"This lady's wearing a light blue dress with yellow figures, a flowered hat . . ."

"One minute," whispered producer John Guedel, following us with a clock.

"Because you're slender, you can wear the flowered dress, but a simpler hat, simpler jewelry, simpler gloves, simpler shoes, simpler bag, simpler — simpler . . ."

"Twenty seconds," whispered Guedel.

"Well, Edith, you think she needs fewer accessories," said Art.

Heaven knows what I said! Without Linkletter, I'd never have lived through those first programs. In my panic I talked so fast I was unintelligible. But the women wanted help; most of them hated the way they looked, or their husbands hated it, or their children or their friends. Help them I must.

After a while, I became very sure of myself. I acquired so much assurance, I could even be gay. "Oh, lady, less accessories!" I'd say, or "To tell you the truth, your hips *are* too big!" Sometimes our sponsor was a trifle startled. But the women were good sports, no one ever got angry, and in seven years on the air I began to be a cross between Beatrice Fairfax and Emily Post. It was a very "family" program, the patients seemed to enjoy telling me their problems. I was deluged with mail off the air and considered myself quite a wit on.

Then — September 1952 — the program went on television. Talk about learning a lesson! That I was neither young nor beautiful I was well aware; but now a camera was my adversary and I was as paralyzed as a prize fighter by the first punch. When the bell clanged and we took to the air, I wouldn't "fight," I tried to hide behind Art Linkletter. Letters poured in criticizing my clothes, my hats and my dark glasses, especially the dark glasses. And it was true, I wore dark glasses — because, subconsciously, I didn't want people to think I needed to wear glasses at all; I wanted them to think I was wearing sun glasses. "If you're blind, get a tin cup," one letter said. "If not, take 'em off."

Finally, I grew so worried I asked to see a kinescope of the show, *and* I nearly died of mortification! More than my worst fears, worse than in *Lucy Gallant* — there I was looking a little like a big-eyed bug. I was standing wrong, cringing as if I expected Link to hit me over the head. I seriously considered giving up the whole thing. But the program offered me valuable research, and was carrying information to millions of women identifying themselves with our guinea pigs in search of glamour. Did I say millions? Eight and a half millions to be exact, a greater audience than I had ever had, women who'd passed up movie fashions as far beyond them, women who lived in such remote spots they seldom saw a movie — were out there asking us on the Linkletter show for help. I stayed on. And if I was telling others, why not let them tell me? I dropped the dark glasses for the lightest tint that would still let me see under the lights. Every few weeks since September '52, I've faced the world; and, like a surgeon operating in a giant clinic, I've become so absorbed with what is happening that I've gradually relaxed about myself.

One thing I learned early — there is no such thing as a woman who is perfectly satisfied with herself. On screen you have the Magnanis who say, "I am Magnani, I do not wish to change," but in the everyday world almost every woman wants to look different. Not only that — it matters to her vitally. And why shouldn't they change? It isn't too difficult. Very few have anything desperately wrong with them; very few have figures that couldn't be helped with the correct lines. Everyone doesn't have to look like a designer's dream. I say sacrifice style any day for becomingness, for the look that is attractive to *you*.

The majority of women on the Linkletter show have as their weak point a figure defect which they reveal rather than conceal: overweight women, for example, in sleeveless dresses.

"Your upper arms aren't slim," I say. "Wouldn't it be better to cover them?"

"Well, but it's so hot!" And they laugh, sheepishly.

Other women have on too much of everything. They evidently feel that if they are not terribly well dressed, putting on lots of added accessories will help. If one pin is good, four are better.

One half hour before the show, Art Linkletter asks the women in the audience to write their questions on cards. The cards are brought to me, and out of the sixty or seventy I select five with interesting problems, problems which represent a good cross-section. I try to avoid the totally individual problem, and we avoid *men*, although I did answer one cowboy from Montana who wanted to know what to do about bowlegs!

Of them all, through the years, there are several women I remember vividly. . . .

I am dumpy all over [one card said]. My friends are very critical. This is the third time I've come to your program, I thought you could help me.

Dumpy, the card said. . . .

When I finally saw her, I went into a state of shock. How to do this and not hurt her? In such a fragment of time?

Dumpy she certainly was — short, thick and broad in the beam (about 5'3, weight around 150), short-necked, heavy armed. *And dull!* She was wearing a mousy-colored spring dress, chosen to look inconspicuous, a utilitarian dress, three inches too long — evidently to make her appear taller — and pulled in with a wide belt evidently intended to achieve a waistline. The plump arms were bare, the neck covered.

"What is your name?" Art Linkletter was saying. "Please try to speak a little louder. Just a little louder. . . ."

She represented absolutely the way I'd dress an actress to make her look unattractive and heavy on the screen. She'd made herself into such a nondescript, subdued creature she could hardly speak above a whisper.

"What can I do?" she whispered. "I can't get any thinner, I've tried. I'd *like* to look better. Even my husband doesn't like the way I look."

"You could look slimmer wearing a darker color," I said gently but firmly. "I don't mean black — it's summer; but something darker — blue, or charcoal with white accents; and not a wide belt, a narrow belt the same color as your dress. You'd find any two-piece dress more flattering. And wear sleeves to cover your upper arms. Now let's develop the most important thing about you. You have a very pretty, round friendly face."

She blushed and giggled.

"May I try something?" And I quickly unfastened the top two buttons of her dress and turned the neckline down into a V. I took my own scarf, draped it over her plump bare arms, took off her wide belt and lifted her skirt a good three inches. The effect was magic, the audience applauded.

Now you could see her pretty face and neck, you could see her nice feet and ankles; the lower neckline cut the thick look of shoulders and bust. She looked incredibly younger! "The long skirts make you look older, so do the high necks," I told her. "If you wear dark, simple dresses, and frame your face with collars and becoming necklines . . ." All simple, ordinary suggestions she might have culled from any magazine or newspaper. But people don't quite know how to use the information that's available.

"I've always felt so dumpy, so drab, so nothing," she said, forgetting the mike, forgetting Art Linkletter, talking to me as if I were a doctor. When the program was over she came backstage and I made her some thumbnail sketches: necklines, collars, hats.

I never saw this woman again, but a month later she sent me snapshots. "Even my husband notices the change!" she wrote on the back of one snapshot, and she looked very happy.

It must take a lot of courage to get up like that before eight million viewers; it takes courage for me, and I'm a professional; but they come, these women. . . . A crippled teen-age girl, in leg braces, leaning on canes and murmuring:

"Do you think I should dress so people won't notice me?"

"You should dress exactly as though you had nothing wrong with you. You're a very pretty girl. Let's pretend you're a star. With your coloring, wear brighter colors . . ."

"My folks think I should wear dark clothes, plain clothes."

"I say your eyes are your most important feature, and blue should be your most becoming color. Wear it."

. . . A young woman in a wheelchair who said casually, "Clothes mean a lot to me, I want to know how I should look from the waist up." We talked about hats and necklines.

. . . A tall, handsome woman, very long-waisted, who feels she needs high heels, but with high heels is as tall as her husband. I told her when she is with her husband to wear lower heels if that makes him feel more comfortable, and to wear high heels when she's with her women friends and style is more important. Every woman owes it to her husband or escort to dress in a way that will make him feel comfortable.

. . . A charming, dignified woman of thirty-five, probably president of her P.T.A., whose husband makes fun of her because she's bowlegged and who loves to wear pants. There are plenty of costumes less revealing than Capri pants, and I think it unwise to have ridicule, especially from one's husband.

. . . A young woman with a baby in arms who said, "I have an awful problem, the baby keeps grabbing at my hat. He knocks it off all the time." I suggested she not wear the hat. And did that boomerang! At once came letters from milliners insisting I was taking the bread out of their mouths.

. . . A woman, sixty, who wants to look younger because her mother, eighty, looks as young as she does. She was pretty tired of the whole thing, everyone thinking her mother was her sister. What she had on — navy blue dress, white sweater, small white hat — would have been suitable for a woman of any age, twenty-five to fifty-five. Trying to *dress* younger would not make her *appear* younger.

"Why not get Mother to dress older?" suggested Art Linkletter.

We have many variants on the program. Recently we had a contest where several women were given thirty hats, scarves, flowers, jewelry and three minutes to select their accessories. Then I was to tell them right or wrong. We have fashion shows; we talk about clothes; women are selected at random, given a small amount of shopping money; we discuss how they should dress — then they return and I analyze their clothes' selection. Or we pick two or three women who aren't happy with themselves; they come to the studio and let me supervise their dressing; we show them on the program before and after. Most of them can't believe it — can't believe that the changed creatures are themselves! And the "miraculous changes" are simple, really; in many cases, just the matter of not dressing tailored all over or fancy all over. Eye-catchers are important, but a figured dress, a fancy hat, fancy jewelry and fancy shoes are too much.

Always, after the show, we have a small clinic backstage and we cover a good deal more ground than we were able to cover in the few minutes on camera. I explain that the first point of emphasis is shopping. They are inclined to buy impulsively, without relation to things they already have, and they are frequently influenced by what another woman wears. You can't be influenced by anyone, certainly not by the salesgirl (who wants to make a sale) or by the dear friend (who doesn't want to hurt your feelings). Most of these same women are good executives in the way they do their food marketing; they plan ahead, they co-ordinate their purchases and see that nothing goes to waste. Now to do the same thing in fashion terms.

If they've already bought wrong, they are helpless in changing it. Sometimes I can help there, too. During World War II, I did countless advice articles, for materials were scarce and clothes had to be made do. Dresses worn under the arm or in the sleeves can have the sleeves removed and become smart jumpers. Men's frayed shirts can be cut down to make a blouse; necklines can be squared. Suit jackets showing wear can be made into sleeveless cardigans. A jacket can be shortened to bolero length and worn with a gay sash made from an old dress. There are endless tricks. In 1947, one sweep of the designer's pencil outmoded nearly everything in every wardrobe. Women were rebellious, frantic, or both. The Hollywood extra who usually provides her own clothes was as hard hit as the Main Street housewife. At Paramount we remade 600 evening dresses, 400 day dresses, 450 suits, converting them to the new style look for dress extras.

For many a bit player, we transform a star's dinner gown into a handsome negligee or cocktail dress. First aid is something we're just naturally prepared to do for clothes; and the average woman with a budget problem could help herself immeasurably clotheswise by learning how to sew. There are endless ways to doctor dresses, and if you can begin from scratch, make your own clothes, you can really create wonders. Select a pattern; identify yourself with a pattern. In the last few years I've done several designs for the Advance Pattern Company. I'm not allowed to do it commercially; the money goes to charity. I do it because I've found that the Linkletter women wanted patterns!

Many people wonder why we *make* everything worn on screen, buy nothing ready-made. For *Rock-a-Bye Baby*, Jerry Lewis suggested that leading lady Connie Stevens just go out to the store and *buy* something to wear. He didn't want her to have fancy clothes; she was a small-town girl. When we showed Jerry the results of our shopping, he cried, "Make 'em!" Ready-made clothes are made to fit anyone and each individual has figure differences. In making your own clothes, you can adjust to those figure differences, play up your good points, see that the waist fits at the waist, the shoulders are exactly the right width, the darts in the right place.

"What is the length of my skirt supposed to be?" . . . "Would it be better to put plain buttons on this dress?" . . . "Will the current fad last?" . . . "Should I wear it?" . . . The questions backstage at the Linkletter show are simple, but the effect is unlimited.

Did I once dream of turning Hollywood into a place of sleek, beautifully tailored women with the greyhound look? Today I dream bigger. Better than "elegant" to me is AP-PROPRIATE. The message I'm trying to convey on the air is: Look right for the time and place. The cardinal sin is not being badly dressed, but wearing the right thing in the wrong place.

There is a point every woman can learn from the actress. Do your clothes justice — never appear in them *half-baked*, be the finished product. An actress doesn't wear a dress or suit and say, "This'll look wonderful when I have the right shoes and the right hat." She knows that each impression she makes is important, that she's always being seen. She takes pride in herself.

So should we all.

"Oh yeh!" some of you are probably saying. "It's easy to *talk.*"

But I don't just talk, I experiment. And not always on actresses or on the Linkletter show. My very favorite guinea pig happens to be — me.

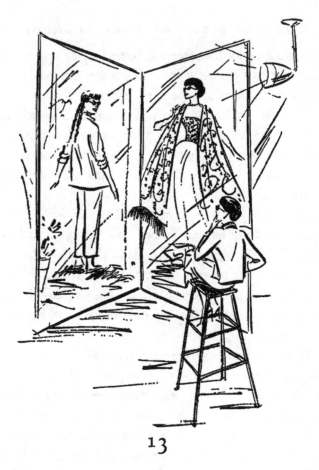

13

My Favorite Guinea Pig — Me

WHEN I BECAME head designer at Paramount and went to
Paris to take on the aura of the *haute couture*, I sailed with
one determination, to change myself completely. I never
had liked the way I looked: my hair, my face, my whole
rather frightened, bespectacled self; here was my chance to

try the magic on me and return a new woman — *Madame* Edith Head.

First, I went to the great hair stylist, Guillaume, and put my head in his hands. It was a short-cropped head, something like Colleen Moore's Dutch flapper bob, and it wasn't important enough for Guillaume. It fell to one of his fifty-seven assistants, who studied it carefully and turned it into a pineapple — bangs swept up, back and sides swept back and up. I believe he called it a coxcomb effect. I couldn't see it too well myself, having just abandoned glasses for a lorgnette.

Then I went to the collections. At Schiaparelli's, I ran into Edward Everett Horton and his mother, and we sat enchanted with the tall, sleek models in their tall, sleek clothes. (If ever there was a designer who catered to height it was Schiaparelli!) Mrs. Horton knew what she wanted: a red dress. She found it and ordered it. I didn't know what I wanted; I'd already purchased suits and tailored clothes; now I wanted the Madame Edith dress. It appeared, finally, on a model at least six feet tall (it should have stayed on her), a black dinner suit embroidered in pink and yellow sequins with long lemon-colored gloves worn to the shoulder. This was for me, even though it cost a fortune. Because of the embroidery it cost me another fortune going through Customs; but it was worth every cent. I arrived home, locked myself in, tried on the new gown, the new hair-do and the lorgnette — and never to this day has anyone else ever seen "Madame Edith"! If the effect was awful the experience was most salubrious and taught me a lasting lesson. The creature who faced me in the mirror was not *me*. I hung the dress away in the closet (it's still there), put on my glasses, combed my own hair and decided who I was.

Not that you can have only one style. Let me refute that idea quickly. Style is just as important for you as it is for your home, your car, and so on. I experiment. I don't say, "I can wear only beige suits with white collars" (my favorite); I follow fashion. I couldn't expect my distinguished clientele to pay me much heed if I didn't. Besides, the emotional power of clothes is terrific; they are the best nerve medicine in the world; why not use them?

I experimented. I'm not a bad guinea pig, either. I'm just over five feet, I couldn't be accused of being a grey-hound, but that is no reason for being negative. I don't look like anyone else. Why should I? That was a mistake that held me back for a long time: *trying* to look like other people. Then, about twelve years ago, I began concentrating on me and evolved a style of my own. Colors overpowered me, prints overpowered me, so, be monotone.

Every woman has at least two personalities. As a dress de-signer I allow myself several. At work, to be background, I wear the tailored suits, the softly tailored dresses, usually in monotone colors. (Right now, in spring, I'm wearing three suits, all the same style: one in linen, one in tweed, one in camel's hair, with coats, one long, one short, one medium, all in shades of pale wheat. I might add that even though these suits are tailored, they are high fashion, and they achieve what I want: individuality.) For great occasions, I wear very extreme evening clothes — my favorite, at the moment, a white embroidered cotton (the material came from Switzerland) with a flared skirt slim at the top and very full at the bottom, and a short jacket bordered in black sable. At home I dress in a casual fashion (usually white or natural homespun). At the moment I'm having made a series of off-white skirts with unpressed pleats, interchangeable tops with push-up sleeves and varied necklines. On a Saturday morning at Casa Ladera (the house on the side of the hill), you'd probably find me playing with my cats or gardening in the patio in a pair of white peon pants and a boxy jacket of the same stuff.

One thing for sure, at home no one would know I'm a career woman. Perhaps this is because I don't particularly *like* career women: I think they can be treacherous animals to live with; they often take their careers too big — the working part of their lives eclipses their private lives. I've designed wedding finery for many a lovely romance that didn't last, perhaps because the women were too competitive, because they were so submerged in their careers and the competition involved. It's very tiring to be with people who are unremittingly competitive. These girls are very successful careerwise, but they're no longer married; they forgot to turn off business when they came home. Other competent career women *are* successful at work *and* in marriage, but they couldn't be married to Bill (Wiard) Ihnen. No one could be an executive at home and be married to Bill.

And that's the man to whom I'm married. He was born in this country, but he lived in Europe a great deal, and he has the European point of view about being head of the house. It's an interesting point of view, and I not only respect it, I like it.

Wiard Ihnen came to Paramount about the same time I did (no one could pronounce his name so we all called him "Bill"). We grew up together on the lot, and occasionally worked together on pictures (as an Art Director, Bill has two Oscars of his own). We became close friends from the time we worked on *The Cradle Song*, lunched together, and were completely compatible. If he forgot to ask me at lunch, he'd often phone me later: he was taking some girl to the opera that night, what flowers should he send? Or he was taking someone to a concert, and she was wearing a red dress, what kind of corsage should he send?

I didn't tell him that I personally don't wear corsages, that unless a dress is specifically designed to demand a corsage, it's a superfluous ornament. *Carry* flowers, yes — use a sprig of flowers in a suit lapel; or at night, if you're the Grace Kelly type, a rose in your hair. I didn't give Bill a dissertation, I just told him what to send. I always liked him. He is a great artist and has great taste, extraordinary taste (except in corsages).

Then one time his good friend, Victor Calderón, came on a visit from Spain and the night he arrived we all had cocktails together.

"You two have been going together a long time, when are you going to get married?" Victor asked.

"He hasn't asked me," I said.

"Tomorrow," Bill said.

"Fine, I'll arrange everything." And Victor raised his glass *To the Ihnens.* "We'll pick you up tomorrow morning."

I had no idea whether he was serious or not. I did *not* don bridal finery. As a matter of fact, I put on a hot red-and-yellow hand-woven dress and a big straw sombrero. That certainly looked casual.

Bill showed up bright and early bearing the biggest purple orchid in the world; and my feeling for floral décor notwithstanding, I promptly pinned it to my hot red and yellow bosom. Evidently we were getting married. We drove to the airport, and Victor and Bill ushered me to a tiny chartered plane, the smallest plane I'd ever seen, and introduced me to the pilot. I'm afraid of BIG planes! This one held four people neatly packed, but the pilot asked if he might bring along his girl friend and we didn't have the heart to say no. Somehow the little plane was airborne and headed east. The pilot radioed ahead to have a taxi meet us and we trundled into Las Vegas. Then he dropped us off at the Golden Nugget while he went to see about getting us a judge.

I couldn't resist the sounds of jingling coin. I got some silver dollars, advanced on the roulette wheel and put a silver dollar on number four.

"You don't put your money on a number," Bill said. "You work out a system." At that moment number four came in and paid thirty-five dollars. Bill couldn't stand it, he walked away — because this time I put all thirty-five dollars on four. It worked just fine. I'd never won a dollar in my life before or since, but I couldn't lose that day, and it was quite a pile by the time the pilot and his girl friend came back to say they'd found a judge.

This was September 8, 1940. I must confess that we did not live "happy ever after." Our first year of wedded bliss was somewhat impeded by two complete sets of furniture. I was living on Doheny Drive at the time, in a house full of dainty French provincial furniture; it looked, really, a little like a French house of ill repute. Bill had a house on Sunset Plaza filled with authentic Mexican and Spanish furniture. When he was a very young architect, he read a book called *The Bible in Spain* and he and another young painter promptly took off for "Mecca." He fell in love with Spain, actually, and in return trips collected many wonderful things.

We bought our first house and moved in to it all my dainty French furniture and all Bill's massive Spanish. The two languages didn't mix. We were both totally stubborn. Our possessions were highly stylized, we loved them, we weren't about to give. After a year, the message finally came through to me that Bill was the architect and I was the dressmaker. Very quietly, I got rid of all my furniture except that in my bedroom. It is still French provincial, the covering of my French daybed red-and-white toile de Jouy.

And of course it was Bill who found our present home and talked me into it: a Spanish Colonial house, California style. (If that sounds complicated, it is. Bill says that when New England sea captains came down to Mexico and California to get hides, they brought along shiploads of doors, windows, window frames, etc. They used these for ballast and barter and introduced into Spanish architecture the double hung windows and paneled doors of New England.) In any event, the place was charming, Bill told me; it had walls four feet thick, a *galería*, and, sweeping up behind the *galería*, a mountainside covered with greenery. He'd fallen completely in love with it.

"When you see it, Edith, don't obviously like it too much," he said. "I've already gone overboard and the agents and the owner know it. Of course if you don't like it, we'll just forget it." With that he tucked me in the car and we *rushed* right over. It looked like an authentic Mexican hacienda to me, a little austere (it wasn't landscaped then, as Bill later landscaped it); and the man who had built it years before had loved heavy substantial construction, had been meticulous about every detail that contributed to his comfort, including a steam bath — but he had omitted closets altogether. Four and a half acres of land, a forty-square-foot steam bath, no closets.

I objected loudly. Bill had said, "Don't be too enthusiastic" — I objected, too, to the huge arch in the living room; I didn't like the baronial fireplace, and the steps leading to the breezeway were trimmed in blue tile. Blue is not my favorite color, I'm the lime-yellow type. We went back home.

"Well, that's that," Bill said. "I guess it was too big, anyway; there'd have been a lot of work; I've begun to hate it myself." He looked very grave, one finger rubbed across his black mustache. (He has a very fierce mustache.)

"But Bill, that's what you *told* me to do!"

"You mean you *liked* the house?"

"Yes, it's a lovely house, it's just that I don't like blue tile and there aren't any closets."

"You fooled me," Bill said. "You overacted. Let's buy it." And a gleam came into his eye. "I'll remake it."

Before the day was over, we'd bought it. I traded in my chic sophisticated French housecoats for the homespun that goes with Casa Ladera. Not that I wander around looking like a Mexican refugee. I never wear pure Mexican, I do derivations; and I'm enough of a ham actress to know that Bill, in selecting the type of architecture, the structure and massiveness he liked, also gave me the most flattering background I could possibly have. I feel I look as if I might have been born on the place. He built me a dressing room any movie star would envy, a whole room paneled from top to bottom in drawers.

He has also built another wing to the house, plenty of closets, and some of the most magnificent furniture I've ever seen; and we've had a wonderful time collecting the Mexican tin masks, the pottery and copper we use for decorations (one wall of the cantina is covered with Mexican hats, there are hanging copper pots in the open kitchen at the far end of the patio, and fresh flowers before the small shrines.) Best of all is the atmosphere of peace and ease, and not the least in establishing this atmosphere, Nannie, who has kept house for me for twenty-one years. This is another world, where studio problems don't exist. They shouldn't exist. I learned long ago to block out and bury things I don't like, things that hurt. I have in my mind a special room with iron doors. The things I don't like I throw in there and slam the iron door. Occasionally, when I do bring a problem home, Bill and I talk it out. He knows the studio, he worked there for years; we speak the same language. He's practising architecture now and painting, something he's always wanted to do. He knows how to *use* time, and our week ends are vacations — barbecuing, swimming, playing tennis, doing things around the house we both love. And of course, caring for the cats. They are Miguel and Minerva (Spanish for Mickey and Minnie Mouse), brother and sister, and hate each other with an unparalleled hate. We even feed them separately; we pretend there's only one cat at a time. I love animals as I did when I was a child. Bill laughs at me, carrying caterpillars out of the house and putting them back in the earth, or warning him away when the snails come out on the ivy in the evening: "Don't step on him, Bill, he has an important date over there on that geranium."

Bill likes to garden, I love to cook. My mother was an excellent international cook, I still use her recipes; and when we travel, I bring back new specialties, dishes we've eaten and liked; I record them automatically in this funny photographic head of mine, with what goes in them. From this last trip, spaghetti with clams from Italy, and salade Niçoise from the south of France; from Spain a cold vegetable soup, *gazpacho*.

Cooking was my "category" on the Groucho Marx show. (That surprised them!) And how I boned for that exam"! I knew the questions would be erudite, so I memorized *The Gourmet Cookbook* (in toto), some Mexican and French cookbooks, etc. I went through wines and sauces. Then I hit the show. Question I: "What is a Kentucky Wonder?" That was easy: a bean. I waited for the double-cross. "What is the name of a famous breakfast dish served in Philadelphia made of pork and meal fried together?" Easy: Scrapple. Question Three: "What are crêpes Suzette?" Easy. The French pancakes. Then the jackpot question: "What famous statue is among the seven wonders of the world?" That was the Colossus of Rhodes. I won, of course, two thousand dollars; but Bill will never let me live down the week I spent memorizing cookbooks.

I should have taken baseball as a subject. If I ever go on again (and I won't), I'll take my favorite sport. I never knew about baseball until we made *Rhubarb*, the story of a cat who inherited a baseball team. As a lover of cats, even ornery ones, I felt it my duty to investigate the sport to which he was addicted, and I've been a mad fan ever since. Oh, those Milwaukee Braves! I'm probably the one dress doctor in town who can identify a fungo fly.

The designing business takes you into strange fields. Remember for a long time I thought of ducking the whole issue and returning to schoolteaching? Well, when I did go back to teaching, the subject was "Motion Picture Costume De-

sign," the school was UCLA, and the students were Marines,
soldiers and sailors on the G.I. Bill. I thought they were ac-
credited students and could draw. They thought I could
put them in touch with the popular pin-up girls. It was a
great case of mistaken identity. I'd taught school twenty
years ago when teachers were teachers and students students.
Progressive methods have evidently changed all that, because
they did not treat me like a venerable professor.

But like a venerable professor I am treated in many unexpected places. Two years ago, when Bill and I arrived in
Germany on vacation, Paramount International mentioned we
were coming and it took us three hours to get out of the airport. In addition to radio and news reporters and photog-
raphers, there was a young newspaperwoman who sat me
down to design a blouse "suitable for *all* German women."
That is covering quite a lot of territory: the shorts, the talls,
the fats, the thins. I sat down and designed a wraparound
blouse. . . . In Holland, I found myself facing 350 Dutch
women who had assembled to find out what *they* should wear,
and I tried to tell them via an interpreter. . . . In the Japanese section of town, here, recently, we were buying in-
gredients for sukiyaki. A Japanese mother who could not
speak English had her daughter ask, Wasn't I from the Linkletter show? And should Japanese-American women wear
American clothes or Japanese clothes here in America?

I suggested: "American clothes for street wear, but by all
means keep your lovely kimonos for home wear. They're
beautiful, they suit you and you love them."

In a motor court at Nogales last Christmas vacation, we came out of our room to find a delegation from Oklahoma — mother, father, aunts, grandma and a very heavy teen-age girl. Wasn't I the lady from the Linkletter show? What was wrong with the way this girl looked? While Bill packed the car, I suggested that instead of a plaid skirt, she try a solid dark color; instead of the bright, tight sweater, a flannel blouse. . . . In Gila Bend, when we stopped for a beer at a little roadside restaurant, we leaned our elbows on the counter with the truckdrivers, drank our beer, and glanced at the newspaper. The front page described the wedding of THE BRIDE OF THE YEAR, a Gila Bend girl in a white satin gown with "the famous *Sabrina* neckline."

On this trip through the desert, incidentally, we stopped at a small store; I bought Christmas ornaments, and, out in the middle of nowhere, decorated a little greasewood tree. For the moment, time slipped away; so did the world of fashion, and I remembered a long-ago pigtailed girl toying with bits of greasewood under the desert sun. If a burro had shown up, I'd probably have taken off my own silk scarf and resumed business as usual.

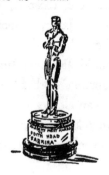

APPENDIX

For the Do-It-Yourself
Dress Doctor

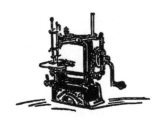

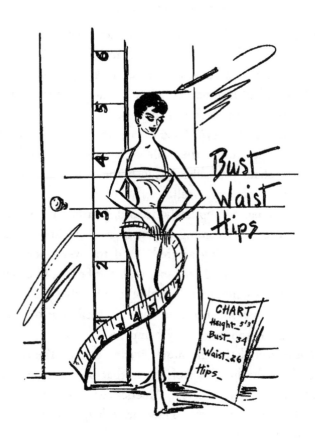

CHART
Height 5'3"
Bust 34
Waist 26
Hips

What Clothes Can Do for You

OBVIOUSLY, THIS IS a far more complex subject than can be dealt with in three quick minutes on television. Clothes have to do with happiness, with poise, with how you *feel*. You never forget the dress or suit in which you looked well, felt right, and lived wonderful moments — the "Alice Blue

Gown." Grace Kelly felt drab, dull and downbeat in her *Country Girl* sweater, the clothes depressed her. Anna Magnani felt slovenly and miserable in her sack slip. From Charles Laughton to Yul Brynner, costume has helped immeasurably with every role an actor has to play.

Why wouldn't they? Clothes are the way you present yourself to the world; they affect the way the world feels and thinks about you; subconsciously they affect the way you feel and think about yourself.

If you are not appropriately dressed, you lose the essential importance of all grooming — you lose the feeling of being comfortable and feeling assured. And for every moment of a woman's life, within her home, with her family, in business if she's a professional person, feeling comfortable and assured are exactly what she needs to feel. It spells the difference between poise and inferiority complex.

That correct clothes are much needed therapy I've come to realize from the hundreds of letters that pour onto my desk weekly, from women across America who are deeply dissatisfied with themselves. They need help and hope, and both are available.

Every woman, like every actress, is capable of being visually translated into many different women. A woman in a bathtub has little personality, she's just a woman without clothes. Clothes not only can make the woman — they can make her serveral different women. There's no one style, there's a style for a mood: a tailored woman at work, a siren at night, a feminine, attractive creature at luncheon, an efficient chairman of a P.T.A. meeting. Working wives must cultivate two separate fashion philosophies: no man wants a brisk, executive-looking woman at the dinner table, and no man wants a too-alluring creature gliding around his office.

I remember a picture in which Irene Dunne played a rich woman with a great feeling about women's place in the world, international affairs, and such. She needed to look beautiful and intelligent. "I don't want to look like a businesswoman," Irene said. "But I do want to look like a woman a man would talk to." I put her in dark silk with white at wrist and throat, lovely millinery. Recently, at a fashion show, I ran into Irene, now a delegate to the United Nations. She was wearing a dark silk dress, the most feminine white hat I'd ever seen, white gloves and pearls. She looked exactly like a woman a man would talk to.

Good clothes are not a matter of good luck. They are a result of thorough knowledge of the person you are dressing: her measurements, her coloring and facial contours; and, even more important, what makes her tick. Clothes counterbalance personality, play it up or play it down. Each woman's task is to be a do-it-yourself dress doctor, and the person she must know is herself.

The questions to ask are:

WHO AM I? . . . WHAT DO I WANT TO CONVEY?

STEP 1: *Let's analyze your figure.* At the studio, I put an actress into a skin-tight straight jacket of heavy white muslin and fit it tightly to her figure. This gives me an exact picture of her figure, its faults and good points, what should be emphasized, what minimized.

At home, stand before a full-length mirror in either a bathing suit or your briefest underwear. Look at yourself from the neck down and force yourself to be objective. With a tape measure, measure your three major figure points: bust, waist, hips. Stand against the door, mark your height. (Height and measurements — not weight — determine your clothes figure.) Or, tape a large piece of wrapping paper against the wall. Mark your height on it, and your outline, and you'll have an actual figure to look at. *Figures don't lie.*

SHORT? TALL? FAT? THIN? AVERAGE? WELL PROPORTIONED?

These are the facts you must face before you decide what to do with yourself. *You can be smart and attractive no matter what the figure:* the trick is to know your figure and select clothes for *that* figure, clothes that will complement and camouflage whatever the problems are. So let us look at a few popular problems:

TOO HEAVY?

First rule for you: *Don't fit your clothes too tightly.* The tighter the fit, the more apparent the bulk. Wear darker colors, not always black or navy, but dark, medium tones rather than pastels or very bright colors. Be careful of prints and patterns. Prints should be small designs against a darker background; polka dots should be very small, stripes vertical, and the fabrics you choose should have dull surfaces, not shiny. These specific suggestions will help you make the *least* of yourself:

NECKLINE: V, open shirt collar, or narrow square.

BUSTLINE: Slight fullness over the heavy bust is good camouflage. So are narrow revers or collars on a V neckline. Narrow, vertical tucks are good to minimize width, too; and avoid glittery or eye-catching fastenings, large buttons, pins, brooches or long necklaces.

SHOULDERS: Keep them smooth: no padding, no detail.

WAIST: Keep it inconspicuous, with a narrow belt same color as your dress, preferably of same fabric, with a fabric-covered buckle.

ARMS: Uncovered are dangerous when you're plump. Your most flattering sleeve length is below the elbow.

HIPS: Wear your skirts hanging loosely from the waist and don't let them cup below the hips. Your skirt can be straight, gored or pleated. Avoid the gathered skirt, it's treacherous, so are full petticoats.

LEGS: Wear medium dark hose and plain footwear. Fancy shoes just call attention to too-heavy legs. If you have dainty legs and feet, which many heavy women do, be as gay as you wish.

SILHOUETTE: Your most flattering silhouette is *any version of the two-piece garment:* suit, or dress and jacket. The two-piece look is flattering because the loose jacket hides heaviness through the middle. An overblouse is another good bet. If you want a one-piece dress, choose one that opens down the front with a fold or piping to emphasize this line; it breaks the width of your figure.

COATS: Let them fit easily and be simple in cut. Avoid big collar and cuffs, avoid heavy revers, avoid too-bulky fabric. If color contrast with your dress is wanted, wear your dress in the darker shade, your coat in the lighter. If your coat is less than full length it must be of the same color value as your dress.

FURS: The short-haired furs are your best friends. (This includes mink!) In a stole, select short-haired fur in the darker shades, straighter lines. Fur scarves (four, five or six-skin) are very becoming to you. In selecting a fur coat, avoid anything shorter than hip length. Full length is preferable. Fur-trimmed coats are attractive, especially when fur is used in tuxedo fronts or in narrow collars.

ACCESSORIES: Most heavy women have pretty faces, pretty throats, chests, wrists and hands. Concentrate on them. Use interesting collars, scarves and jewelry. If you have pretty wrists, use cuffs and bracelets. Wear earrings by all means (not too large or too bulky) and in necklaces avoid chokers and select a graceful medium length. Hats are where you can really go to town! Your face is your fortune? Frame it.

TOO THIN?

Can you imagine slenderness being a problem? From the fashion point of view, of course it isn't. However, there are danger areas. The woman who is slim is likely to have too small a bust, too thin legs, neck, arms and shoulders. First rule for those of you who are too thin: *Don't fit your clothes too tightly.* The tighter the fit, the more glaring the fault. You don't want to look bony. The darker the color, the thinner you'll look. *You* can wear bright colors and pastels, and white and bold patterns; you can wear any fabric that you wish. To make the *most* of yourself watch . . .

NECKLINE: High necks are safest but you can use a lower neckline by filling it with soft scarves, jewelry or bows. For a more uncovered look, try sheer yokes the color of your dress or yokes of nude net. Try wide, flat costume jewelry or several strands of pearls to cover collarbones. Fortunately, the covered-up look is very smart, and you don't have to feel you're concealing anything.

BUSTLINE: In selecting a padded bra, be careful to select one in proportion to your frame, a large bust on a slender chassis can look grotesque. If you don't care to use padding for the fuller look (and I very seldom do in pictures), use fabric fullness, gathers or soft pleats. Loosely fitted blousetops are good, too. Lighter material than that used below the waist will make you look larger, so will patterned fabric.

WAIST: Thank your lucky stars and accentuate it with wide belts, contrasting colors, cummerbunds, sashes and interesting buckles.

ARMS: Cover them with full (not tight) sleeves. Cuffs add interest and flattery at the wrist; they're excellent bone concealers.

HIPS: *If* you feel your hips are too slim (possible?) wear gathers, pleats or peplums.

LEGS: Light hose, preferably seamless, will become you best. And do not wear shoes that contrast too greatly with the color of your hose. Keeping leg and foot close in color value reduces the chance of your legs' looking too thin. Full skirts help too.

SILHOUETTE: You can wear the most extreme styles: tight waists, full skirts and petticoats, the draped, the sheath, the tunic, the peplum, the shirtmaker dress and any version of the two-piece dress. If you like sweaters and are very thin, try twin sweaters, undersweater plus cardigan, and possibly a scarf.

COATS: Select what you will — slim, wraparound, voluminous or belted, flat or bulky material in any color.

FURS: Stoles can be any size, any color, short- or long-haired. Coats can be any length from bolero down. Fur-trimmed coats as extreme as you wish.

ACCESSORIES: Wear costume jewelry so long as it's not *too* heavy. Scarves, bows, ascots are all good. Hats should not be too high-crowned or narrow-brimmed. Veiling is flattering.

TOO TALL?

This, again, is hardly a problem fashionwise. It's really up to you — do you want to accentuate or minimize your height? Obviously if you wish to look shorter, don't wear high heels. There are smart heels in medium heights as well as flats. A two-tone color scheme is important. Try a light top and a dark bottom or vice versa, using the light color where you are more slender, the dark color where you are too heavy. (If you are a tall woman and heavy, you'll want to combine these formulas with formulas for the heavy woman.) If you wish to minimize your height watch these danger areas:

BUSTLINE: Do not emphasize.

SHOULDERS: Do not pad.

WAIST: Emphasize your normal waistline with a color-break — a belt as wide as you wish if your waist is small.

ARMS: No very short sleeves; preferable length, medium. Deeper armholes are an excellent camouflage.

HIPS: Flared skirts, softly pleated or gored skirts minimize height.

LEGS: Don't wear your skirts too short; keep them in relation to your leg.

SILHOUETTE: The two-piece height-breaker is your best choice: skirt and jacket, skirt and overskirt, skirt and tunic or peplum. Full skirts and wide belts are good. Jackets are good; they can be any length.

COATS: Hip length or three-quarter length is preferable; belted coats are very good. Flared coats are very good. Try a contrasting color in your coat, try extreme collars and cuffs.

FURS: Stoles, scarves and jackets are good height-breakers. Wear what you wish, long or short hair. In fur coats, you can wear any length; hip length or three-quarter length are good. On a fur-trimmed coat, avoid the tuxedo front, but fur cuffs, pockets or collars are fine.

ACCESSORIES: Medium or broad-brimmed hats are good for you, so are flat crowns. Use hats for color contrast and avoid the too elaborate. As for jewelry, follow your whim; you have the height to carry even the bulkiest.

TOO SHORT?

The first principle for the small woman is the use of *one color*. Never cut the body line, keep your lines vertical, your prints small, your heels high (except with sports clothes or slacks), and, unless you're under twenty, keep away from the too, too little-girl look. There's no reason why you can't achieve glamour and sophistication in clothes; just be careful they don't overpower you. First principle in designing for a star is never to let the dress overwhelm the personality. This goes for you, too, and one way to insure it is not to call attention to bust, waist or hips.

NECKLINE: Very best, the V. The open shirt collar is good too.

BUSTLINE: Minimize your bustline to avoid looking top-heavy. If you are large-busted, wear no extra ornamentation, no glitter jewelry or buttons in this area.

SHOULDERS: No fullness at the shoulders, no padding, no detail.

WAIST: Omit belts or use narrow belts, self-color or fabric, no heavy pockets, no horizontal trim.

ARMS: Slim sleeves.

SILHOUETTE: Avoid too-long dress length; choose a length that is right in relation to your leg. The slim look is the most rewarding for you; eschew voluminous skirts and petticoats, avoid tunics and peplums. *Keep it simple.*

COATS: The straight coat is best. Avoid the flared coat with heavy collars and cuffs, avoid big buttons and big pockets, avoid bulky fabric.

FURS: Wear them, but keep the furs small, short-haired, small-collared. Be very careful of the fur-trimmed coat — it should have very small collar, narrow revers down the front, small cuffs.

ACCESSORIES: Hats, bags, jewelry — all should be small, to scale. In the matter of shoes, indulge your little feet.

Mrs. Alfred Hitchcock is a very chic example of what clothes can do for the short woman. She has an excellent figure, in perfect proportion; but she's 4'11, according to her passport, and when she walks into a store to buy clothes she's very likely to be shown something suitable for a twelve-year-old girl. Size 8's are seldom sophisticated, and most size 8's don't have to be presented to the Queen of England. Alma Hitchcock, traveling constantly with her famous husband, must look smart and sophisticated; she has the wardrobe problems of a diplomat's wife, and she dare not look too glamorous — the clothes would overpower her. She must be patient, and when she buys clothes ready-made have them scaled down.

Her well-dressed look is based on wearing slim one-piece clothes (she could look dumpy if her clothes were cut in too many places) and on not breaking the line with color or wide belts. She wears jackets, but they match the dress and,

short or long, they're very slim. Of course, she carries herself tall, with a confidence, a poise and a charm that makes
her seem considerably taller. She knows who she is; she
found out fairly early in life how she wanted to look; and
she's worked out her format.

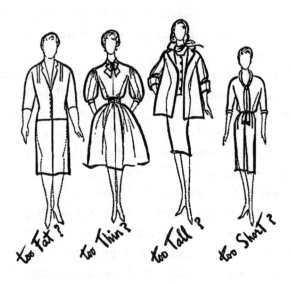

STEP II: *Prepare to go shopping.* Each of us can do what Alma
Hitchcock has done. Each can look better if — she'll take
the time to analyze her figure, the trouble to choose the
right clothes for that figure and have them properly fitted.
Before you go shopping at all, get the right underpinnings.
There are few perfect figures. The money you spend on cor-
rective undergarments is the most important money you

spend. You're interested in the masculine point of view? I wish you could be with me when a producer calls to say:

"Edith, the clothes are fine. Before we test them, will you please get that actress into a bra and girdle?"

Then I go to her and say: "Don't you think it would be better for the test if you wore a bra and girdle?"

"I never wear them!" she's likely to say. "They restrain my acting."

If she's Anna Magnani or Shirley Booth playing a sloppy woman, then it doesn't matter. If she's trying for glamour, then, thanks to the producer, she ends up correctly sheathed. By all means, when you go out to shop for clothes, wear the right girdle, the right bra and the right shoes. Never shop simply because you have "nothing to do." Never buy anything as a whim. In short . . .

STEP III: *Make clothes a business.* Make up your mind what you need. Seasons overlap, and you can't generalize. You have to ask yourself how abrupt the seasons are, how different, and whether or not you can afford them. The young actresses who come to me for help usually bring along all the clothes they have. We lay them out around the room and decide which can go on into spring (or fall), what accessories will go with what (we make a list of accessories which will change the clothes from day to day), what basic clothes they need. You don't buy one dress, or one pair of shoes or one hat unrelated to the rest of your clothes. You plan for a span of time, just as you plan food menus and shop for staples. Then make a "grocery list" and know exactly what you're looking for. This will keep you from squandering your budget on haphazard accessories or a cute hat that matches nothing. Be sure that any item you purchase — from a pair of gloves to a winter coat — helps to give the impression you want to give, will serve you on a number of occasions and be friendly with other items in your wardrobe. We can't all live in penthouses or winter in Florida. What you buy must suit your income and environment.

And don't let anyone tell you that what you have to spend isn't important. It is. The young starlets with their limited budgets would be quite mad to go out and buy white fox capes, even on time, or dresses for a hundred and fifty dollars. They must buy a simple dress that looks elegant, and have enough left for the accessories that dress it up or down. You can buy wonderful clothes inexpensively. Marlene Dietrich was so enchanted with the little six-dollar box jackets she found on Spring Street that she brought one back for every girl in the department. She brought back some charming inexpensive hats, too.

The economic problem is a pressing one, not because clothes aren't available, but because a great many women who have homes to care for, a number of children and a limited budget don't have the time to spend on self-grooming. The first article I ever did on clothes was for *Redbook*, and I did it in the grand manner, with starlets in lovely clothes showing how to look well-groomed and well-dressed while going through the day's routine at home. I was pretty unrealistic about the whole thing, and the readers let me know it. "Miss Head evidently doesn't keep house" . . . "Miss Head evidently has no children . . ." and so on and on.

STEP IV: *Going shopping.* I'm a realist now, and I know that time is a frantic thing for the homemaker without help, and for the working wife, and for the career girl. I can only say, time is an urgent problem of mine, too. The more urgent the time, the more important to make that shopping time count. Having analyzed your figure and your budget, you can give the salesgirl a cue. "I'm broad-hipped. I don't want a full skirt. I do want a two-piece dress for afternoon wear, and let's keep it dark. Also let's keep it inexpensive." Know what you want; when you try it on, be objective. Most of the women I have seen who needed help the most looked as if they had bought their clothes without ever glancing in a mirror. If it were possible to have a Polaroid camera along, snap your own picture and develop it at once, you'd make fewer mistakes. If you haven't a camera, train your eye.

Look at the costume on *you,* not on someone else. How it looked in the style show at lunch doesn't matter unless your measurements and type resemble the model. Be sure that the length is right for your height. I never go to extremes on dress length. (In pictures, I can't. It takes some six months or longer from the time clothes are designed until the picture is released.) I wear my own skirts twelve to fourteen inches off the floor come hell or high waistlines. It's the best proportion for my height and my legs.

Don't buy what is the "last word" or very high-style, or anything bizarre or unusual, if you have to wear your clothes for the next year. Nothing is deader than last year's high style.

Don't buy clothes that do not belong in your life: suit your shopping to your activities.

Buy as many separates or two-piece costumes as you can. They are the salvation of any girl or woman on a budget and will never go out of style.

Look at newspaper ads and magazine ads. Identify yourself with illustrations that resemble you, and look for the type of clothes that seem to become them (we'll talk more about the LOOK you want later).

STEP V: *Don't worry about your age.* If you feel dowdy, you'll certainly look it. If you feel elderly, you'll look that. The almost universal desire of American women is to look YOUNGER. I stress "American," because European women are not similarly concerned; the youth fetish is strictly *our* national anthem. In most women's minds, being young is synonymous with being attractive, romantic, glamorous, having a good figure — all the things that make a teen-ager long to grow up. "Middle age" signifies the exact reverse. Even some actresses show a mounting tension as they approach the dividing line. It depends, actually, on how good an actress is. The good actress is sure of herself; for her youth doesn't have the same desperate emphasis.

The fact is that many of the most attractive, most glamorous women in the world are not young. They have, rather, a sure knowledge of themselves; they are poised, beautiful and adjusted to life; they don't remotely suggest Whistler's Mother. Ethel Barrymore looks like a queen, Dietrich and Swanson have become all-time symbols of glamour. Some women are middle-aged at thirty, some are not middle-aged at sixty. And so far as clothes go — today's American clothes have a young look, they're adaptable to fifteen or fifty-five. It's no longer a matter of age, it's a matter of figure. I know a number of women forty-five who look twenty-five. And they don't achieve this look by wearing girlish clothes (ruffles, pinafores), but by wearing clothes that are ageless: the shirtmaker dress, the sweater and skirt, the suit, the simple dress with crisp collar, sports clothes, pretty colors and fabrics. Obviously young clothes make an older person look older. The point is not how old or how young clothes are, but how well they suit you. Divorce yourself from styles that do *not* suit you, even though your soul yearns for them.

The objective is to make you look glamorous, and by glamour we mean: *accentuate the positive; eliminate the negative.*

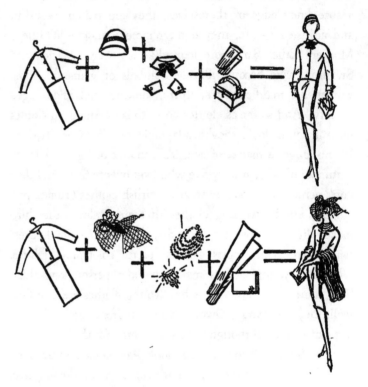

What You Can Do for Clothes

ONCE YOU HAVE bought your clothes, be kind to them, *take them to the right places.* A sun suit may look fine in the sun, but it looks dreadful indeed at the supermarket. You seldom see a badly dressed woman at a sports event. High-heeled satin pumps and tennis shorts went out with Clara

Bow, and women who go to golf meets or football games, or who play sports actively themselves, usually look pretty well. And you seldom see a badly dressed salesgirl. Each store has regulations; salespeople help set up standards of good taste. The danger zones are in the area of too casual public dressing, too dressed-up occasions, and in the area of white-collar jobs.

I don't believe in a hundred rules. They dull a woman's native creativity. Half the fun of being a woman is to experiment with the way you look; but work hours are not the time to decide between Circe and Eloise. Evening is the time. For fun at a party, you can plan whether you want to try for the seductive look (long earrings, sheer black stockings, extreme hairdo) or whether you want the feminine, chiffon-organdy look.

There is no such thing as a healthy woman over the age of five who doesn't enjoy experiment. I can remember my mother at seventy-six, about to go out with friends, saying, "Now tonight I'm going to try so and so," as excited as a girl. This is wonderful; it's fun; it's part of femininity, the same quirk that won't let any of us pass a mirror without looking.

But you can also look *too* anything — too Theda Bara or too Scarlet O'Hara or too Diane Varsi. You should never look as if you were going to a costume ball when you're not. You can translate yourself into *many* women, but not *every* woman. The same chassis seldom adapts equally to *femme fatale* and dewy-eyed ingenue. Experiment, for heaven's sake and your own. Find your type, and assert your individuality; but let me suggest a few axioms to keep in mind:

1. *Don't let your clothes be fitted too tightly.* Even a perfect figure looks better if it doesn't resemble a sausage. Figure exaggeration that stresses anatomy to the whistle point is hardly good taste; it's a holdover, really, from an era when glamour was confused with sex. Only bathing suits should "fit tight."

2. *Don't wear a date dress when you're arriving for a day's work* at the office. The dressy dress, the low-necked lacy blouse, the glitter sweater, all of the glitter category belong to after-dark. So do the diamond-studded plastic sandals. If you won't have time to go home and change, carry a large handbag with jewelry, fresh gloves, something for your hair (tiny veils attached to a comb, a bow or a flower); but don't look as if you were going to a party during daytime hours.

3. *Try dressing for men* instead of for women. It's less competitive and a lot safer. Things that women may think too, too cute can scare a male; and the "too, too" look is usually the basis for a woman looking her worst. Men notice a woman first, her clothes second; they dislike any distortion of figure silhouette deliberately devised to be noticed. Waist, bust and hips must be natural. Fit the dress to the girl, not the girl to the dress.

4. *Don't flout convention.* If you are going to a place where it is correct to wear hat and gloves, wear yours.

5. *Don't be too different.* You don't want to dress like the herd, but you don't want to look like a peacock in

a yard full of ducks. If your friends are wearing sport clothes to a luncheon, don't wear an afternoon dress. Being too much an individualist is not being well dressed.

6. *Don't wear strapless dresses, rompers, sun suits or slacks to go shopping.*

7. Ditto — *to go traveling.* If American tourists could hear what the people say all over Europe, Mexico and South America, they'd try for a more covered-up look and they'd certainly wear skirts. There are fortunate girls (usually under the age of fifteen) who look well in tight trousers; but I have seen so many bulging bottoms in Capri pants, shorts, levis and jeans that I've grown positively to dislike the whole trouser family — in public.

8. *Don't feel that when you are going to a party you must look "dressed up"* — a simple dress is safer if there's a question of what to wear, and you will be much more comfortable simply dressed than overdressed.

9. *Don't submerge yourself totally in "smartness."* If your dress is noticed *before* you, it is not a successful dress. It should be a part of you. "Oh what a stunning dress" is no compliment. "How stunning you look" is.

10. *Don't be afraid to wear a becoming costume many, many times.* It's an old-fashioned idea that you must have a new dress for every occasion or party. Even if you have the money to do so, it isn't necessary. The modern approach is to *change accessories.*

Which brings us to what ACCESSORIES can do for your clothes and you. They can achieve a more youthful or a more sophisticated effect, a sport look, a feminine look. Accessories determine the formality of the average dress or suit, furnish the all important eye-appeal. Be kind to your clothes. You wouldn't put mayonnaise on angel-food cake; don't wear evening jewelry on a tennis dress.

Here is what you can do with accessories. Take a basic dress or a suit, dark or any neutral color. Suppose you want to look as young as possible. . . . With the addition of white collar and cuffs, possibly a tie or a bow (if it's a suit, add a white blouse) plus a simple, brimmed hat, plus short gloves, plain pumps, a box bag, you have a costume that is youthful without being deliberately girlish.

The same dress or suit can become a sport outfit by using a beret or sport hat, plus a sport scarf or ascot (with the suit, a sport blouse), a sport belt, pull-on sport gloves, spectator sport shoes and a pouch bag. Your look is now tailored and casual.

Want to look feminine? Try the same dress with a feminine hat, large or small-brimmed to suit your face and height, trimmed with flowers, ribbons, feathers or veiling. Add a soft chiffon scarf caught up at the neck with pin or flower (with the suit add a frilly blouse), plus crushed gloves, matching pumps or sandals. *Voilà!* The look is feminine.

Want to feel sophisticated? Use jewelry on your collarless dress. (With a suit, open the top of the jacket and fill in with jewelry.) Add a dinner or cocktail hat, matching gloves and shoes. Drape yourself in a fur stole; if you can't afford fur there are many handsome synthetics. There you have an evening glamour look!

It isn't so much a question of what clothes you have, it's what you do with them. It's a question, too, of COLOR. Color is the greatest accessory. The young look can happen with a vivid bow and hat. The sport outfit can use a bright beret and blouse, or a gay, striped, figured or plain scarf. The palest of pink, blue, pastel or white makes gloves, blouse and hat more feminine. For sophistication, we usually avoid bright color and concentrate on *one* color with *one* accent: black with only pearls to spike it, light with dark gloves and hat. Color, we find, changes the actress more than the style of dress or suit she wears.

I used to think that when Mae West said, "No green, Honey," or Barbara Stanwyck, "I hate brown," they were being temperamental. There has been so much more research today on color psychology that we know colors affect people physically, emotionally and mentally.

A woman *should* wear colors that make her feel happy, colors that do something for her, colors that make her feel young. No one should wear colors she doesn't like. Incidentally, you don't have to wear *one* color. A young woman wishing to emphasize youth may wear an entire outfit of pink. A more mature woman might wear that same pastel color in her accessories — bag, hat, scarf, to pick up her darker suit.

Color is the most personal point of all fashion. You should

either get help or work out for yourself what is right for you. Black and white are flexible, they can be used for any mood or expression. White can be gay or somber, black can be stimulating or dreary, so I don't include them in this color chart — a chart based on mood and key, in no way scientific, but to date highly successful in my practice.

COLOR CHART

STIMULATING COLORS: (vivid, bright)	Cerise; Scarlet; Orange; Lemon-yellow
RELAXING COLORS: (soft, grayed)	Ivory; Rose Beige; Powder-blue; Sea-green
HOT COLORS: (intense, strong)	Magenta; Flame; Burnt Orange; Electric Blue
COOL COLORS: (pale, pastel)	Lime-green; Apricot; Mauve; Pale Gray
GAY COLORS: (light, bright)	Chartreuse; Rose Pink; Daffodil-yellow; French Blue
SOMBER COLORS: (dark, grayed)	Charcoal; Puce; Mulberry; Sepia

In the past, blondes always wore pastels, brunettes always wore strong colors and redheads never dared touch red or purple. That changed during World War I and never did come back. Redheads use color carefully today only because their own coloring is so flamboyant. Arlene Dahl, Rhonda Fleming, Tina Louise and Susan Hayward with their beauty and their figures must not look too theatrical. You dress them with emphasis on their coloring in pinks (remember when no redhead would dream of wearing it?), mauve and green.

Color can be your friend or foe, one of your very strongest allies in changing your type, enhancing your good points. Yet most people fear it. "I can't wear gray," they'll say — which is ridiculous. They simply cannot wear certain shades of gray. Or they say smugly, "I always wear blue." If you do, you probably look dull. Worst of all is to go overboard on color. Such as when, with a black dress, the woman wears a magenta hat, magenta shoes, magenta gloves, magenta jewelry and a magenta bag. Color shouldn't be repeated more than twice. Dabs of color give an appearance of busyness. It would be better to choose only a magenta hat and keep all other accessories to the color of the dress itself.

It isn't those who spend the most money who are the most smartly dressed. It's those who spend the most time and thought. If, when you go out, you know that your cotume is smart and that you're neatly and securely put together, if you do not feel it necessary to hike your girdle, adjust your straps, pull your stocking seams straight; you have physical and mental poise. You can wear your clothes with grace and pride — with assurance.

And now we're coming to the crux of the matter: the FORMAT. Any woman out of her teens knows whether she is gay or quiet, the feminine or the athletic type. The question is, What do you want to do about that type — emphasize it or change it? Some things are not possible. If you're the Kate Smith woman, you can't look like Jean Simmons. If you were born with straight hair and large bones, it's futile to concentrate on the very feminine Janie Powell look. You can't *change* broad shoulders — but look what Joan Crawford did with hers!

You can be what you want; the problem is, sometimes, to *find* what you *do* want. I've talked, often, to groups of women who looked almost as if they were a regiment: medium-colored women with little dark dresses, little flowered hats and little fur stoles. For me, everything they wore was of good quality, but too well matched, too much of a pattern, too, too plain vanilla. They were the middle-of-the-roaders and they were playing it safe. Women who are not sure take the middle ground: tried (also a little tired)-and-true cut and color; they feel safe. The effect, unfortunately, lacks individuality.

You are a woman with weapons, why not use them? Why be a sheep when you can be a self?

Everyone has a day's work, a career, in home, office or wherever, and why not express your individuality? See how you can best dress for the day's work to give yourself assurance. Life is competitive; clothes gird us for the competition. The woman who knows her type can skip the rest of this chapter; but the woman who does not — who is timid, or not sure — may read on and decide whether she'll be leopard or lamb (you can't be half and half).

Ideas change. I spent the best part of ten years building up the idea that a sensible, efficient tailored suit (with crisp white blouse, of course) was the only garment for a business career girl. Most Hollywood designers did the same. The severe tailored suit got to be a sort of uniform, Hollywood convincing the working girl everywhere that she should be identifiable at more than ten paces. Then, on a trip abroad, I met some European designers. One of them said. "You American women are so sure of yourselves, so self-confident, you make men feel you don't need help or want help. Other women don't give that effect; but American women — the way they dress — frighten men off."

I saw the light. My businesswomen on screen began looking more like women. I don't mean peek-a-boo blouses or a rose between the teeth, but softly tailored dresses, feminine dresses of wool and silk; and I began making suits that didn't look as if they were screaming for two pairs of matching pants.

The too feminine, too businesslike, too anything look becomes a caricature, part of an old screen technique that indicated "I'm a glamour girl" or "I'm a housewife" on the instant. When I went for my job as schoolteacher . . . when I went for my job as sketch artist . . . I caricatured the part. Today you don't wear the mark of your trade. A secretary, a housewife and a designer can dress alike.

Women who don't know what type they are can use self-identification with some person who is much photographed. On television, in magazines and newspapers there are constant illustrations of women of every type, of every age and size. Ads and commercials no longer use just the stereotyped model, they use women who look like *women*. Shop around. Find someone whose looks you like and with whom you can identify yourself. It's the best way I know to find a "look." If you are a feminine woman and want to dress as such, you may select Mamie Eisenhower. If you're more tailored, Claire Boothe Luce. If you're short and vivacious, Gracie Allen.

If you are slim, broad-shouldered, clean-cut, think of yourself in terms of Doris Day. Everything Doris wears, from sports clothes through formal gowns, carries a look of simplicity. She doesn't permit eye-catchers, she doesn't use tricks.

If you are slim and could be very high-styled, think of Audrey Hepburn, who wears exaggerated style and achieves elegance. To be a Hepburn you'd have to study fashion, make it part of your consciousness. It's a cultivated taste — but it's fun. Why look like last year's bird's-nest if you have a flair?

If you're not tall and *are* curvaceous, think in terms of Shirley Booth, who plays various characters on screen, but is one of the best dressed of women, as you know if you saw her on stage in *Desk Set*. She wears only vertical lines; her clothes are slim with open necklines; and she emphasizes color to complement her hair and eyes.

If you are tall and like the patrician look of Grace Kelly, try it. Her clothes have the woman look. She uses flowers as accessories more than anyone I've known, or a colored velvet ribbon tied round her neck to bring out one color in the print of her dress. Always with Grace there is a feeling of freshness and femininity, an understatement of fashion. Crossed white gloves should be her coat of arms. Many women use one identifying accessory that becomes a trademark.

Look at Hedda Hopper and her hats! Everything else is played straight, but Hedda's hats are her eye-catcher, and an effective one. Look at Garbo's sports hats! Other women emphasize shoes, or scarves, or collars.

Actresses have taught me many things. The average actress is interested in *where she's going, whom she's going to meet;* and on this basis selects a costume. An actress checks with her escort to know whether he's wearing a dinner jacket or tweeds. Nothing is unimportant if it adds to her appearance. She'll diet, exercise, forgo desserts, get plenty of sleep, watch her grooming and suffer pain — if it's important to her career. She sees that her clothes are not only smart, but immaculately kept, cleaned, pressed, ready.

And I in turn would give this advice to every actress with whom I work, to every woman who will listen:

(1) *Be dressed for what you are doing.*

(2) *Have the right accessories.*

(3) *Don't wear your clothes too tight.* A dress should be tight enough to show you're a woman and loose enough to prove you're a lady.

I like that last. You can use it for my epitaph.

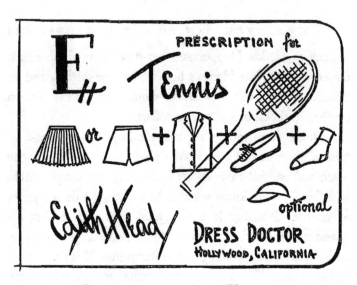

Prescriptions for Dressing

AMUSEMENT PARKS

Spectator sport clothes — skirt + sweater or blouse, or sport dress, sport suit, or simple street dress; + comfortable shoes + sweater or jacket at night. Hat and gloves optional.

ARCHERY

Practice. Shorts, slacks, or action skirt; + shirt + sport shoes + socks + finger tabs and arm guard.

Tournament. White shorts + white T-shirt, or sleeveless blouse, or one-piece sleeveless tennis dress with flared skirt; + white tennis shoes + white socks + white-billed tennis cap + finger tabs and arm guard.

AUTO RACES

Spectator sport clothes — sport dress or sport suit + twin sweaters and skirt, or street dress; + street shoes. Hat and gloves optional.

BADMINTON

Shorts or short skirt + sleeveless shirt, or one-piece action, sleeveless dress (wash fabric, white preferable); + wool ankle socks (white) + tennis or badminton shoes.

Hostess and guests: patio dress or sun dress + patio shoes, thongs or sandals, *or* blue jeans, slacks or shorts, + sports shirt or sweater + flats; or sport dress + sport shoes. For evening barbecues, guests bring sweater or wrap.

BASEBALL

Sport dress, sport suit or skirt + sweater or sport blouse; + comfortable shoes + hat or cap to shade face + gloves if you wish to protect hands from sun. For night games take extra sweater, jacket or coat.

BASKETBALL

Sport suit + twin sweaters and skirt, or sport dress and jacket; + comfortable shoes + topcoat if weather demands. Hat and gloves optional.

BEACH

Bathing suit + beach wrap (coat, cape, pullover or beach towel) + thongs, beach sandals or rope-soled flats. Or shorts, slacks (any length) + halter, sweater or sport shirt, or sun suit, sundress; + beach shoes or flats. Beach hat optional. Beach bag for bathing cap, sun oil, etc.

BEACH RESORT

See VACATION

BICYCLING

Shorts, pedal pushers, or pants, + shirt, sweatshirt or sweater; + sneakers + anklets. Cap optional.

BOATING

Slacks (white duck or light denim) or shorts, + middy, T-shirt, sport shirt or sweater; + cap, hat or hood + *rubber-soled* shoes + windbreaker jacket with or without hood (water-repellent).

Larger Craft. Sport dress, slacks, or shorts with tops mentioned above + overskirt. Take necessary sport clothes for fishing, swimming, etc.

BOAT RACES

Spectator sport clothes in white or light colors — sport dress, sport suit or sport skirt + sport shirt or sweater; + sport shoes + sport hat tightly fitted (it may be windy) + sweater or windbreaker jacket. Gloves optional.

BOAT TRAVEL

See TRAVEL

BOWLING

Slacks, pedal pushers, Bermuda shorts or action skirt, + shirt or sweater; + wool anklets + regulation bowling shoes (shorts permissible but not popular).

BREAKFAST

It's good psychology to start the day with bright colors, so choose something gay in a washable fabric. Breakfast coat, brunch coat, housedress, smock, skirt and shirt or slacks and shirt; + apron if you're cooking; + casual shoes, sandals or flats.

BRIDE

See WEDDINGS, TROUSSEAU

BRIDESMAID

See WEDDINGS

BRIDGE LUNCHEON

See LUNCHEON

BUS TRAVEL

See TRAVEL

BUSINESS* and PROFESSIONAL

City. Suit, or dress + jacket, or day dress, or separates (whole wardrobes can be built with interchangeable skirts and tops); + street shoes + day hat + bag and gloves. A two-piece formula is best for office work, so jacket can be removed. One-piece is best for sales work. Dark clothes with light accents practical.

Country. Sport dress, sport suit, day dress, or separates, in light but not bright colors; + comfortable day shoes.

*Certain professions, of course, require uniforms (nurses, technicians, factory workers, waitresses).

CAMPING

Blue jeans or pants of water-repellent safari-type cloth with cotton or flannel shirt; + sweater + water-repellent jacket + visor cap (optional) + 5 or 9-inch boots (depending on how rough the country) + wool socks. For camp wear, moccasins.

For severe weather. Insulated underwear.

For sleeping. Sweatshirts, such as athletes wear for working out.

CAR TRAVEL

See TRAVEL

CHRISTENINGS

Dressmaker suit or afternoon dress; + afternoon hat + afternoon shoes + gloves. Whether the ceremony is at home or in church, dress as for church.

CHURCH

Day dress, dressmaker suit, or ensemble (dress and jacket); + hat + gloves + street shoes. Hats or head coverings are always correct, in some churches obligatory; bare arms, *incorrect*.

CHURCH WEDDINGS

See WEDDINGS

CIRCUS

Sport suit, sport dress, day dress, dress + jacket. Or skirt with blouse or sweater. Comfortable street shoes. Hat and gloves optional. At night add jacket or coat.

CLUB MEETINGS

Morning. Day dress, or suit; + street shoes + hat + gloves. (*See also* LUNCHEON.)

Afternoon. Dressmaker suit, afternoon dress, or ensemble; + hat + gloves.

Evening. Afternoon dress, or simple cocktail dress, or ensemble; + gloves. Hat optional.

COCKTAIL PARTIES

CITY

Club or Restaurant. Hostess and guests: Dressmaker suit, afternoon dress, cocktail dress, or cocktail suit; + dress shoes + cocktail hat + gloves.

At Home. Hostess: Afternoon dress, cocktail dress, or short dinner dress. Guests: Cocktail suit, cocktail dress, or dressmaker suit (black or dark for winter, pastels or prints for summer); + cocktail or dinner hat + gloves + dinner shoes.

COUNTRY

Country Club. Hostess and Guests: Cocktail suit, cocktail dress, afternoon dress, or dressy sport costume; + dress shoes. Hat and gloves optional.

At Home. Hostess: Sport dress, afternoon dress, or cocktail dress, + dressy shoes. Guests: Sport dress or suit, afternoon dress, or cocktail dress or suit; + dress shoes. Hat and gloves optional.

COLLEGE*

Classroom. Sweater (pullover or cardigan), or blouse (sport or tailored), with skirt (straight, gored, pleated). Or sport dress (shirtmaker, jumper), or sport suit (suitable fabrics — wool, wool jersey, flannel, tweed, cashmere, corduroy; cotton and synthetics in spring); + jacket (cardigan or blazer) + vest + car coat + topcoat + loafers, moccasins, saddle shoes or oxfords + bobbysocks (cuffed) or knee-length socks or hose + gloves (knit or sport) + bag + scarf or hood for campus.

Leisure. Pants — blue jeans to velveteens — Bermuda shorts or pedal pushers; + blouses or sweaters + loafers or leisure shoes.

Social Functions (teas, luncheons). Dressmaker suit or afternoon dress (wool, knit, silk; in spring, prints, cotton, organdy); + jacket or coat + day (not sport) shoes + hose + small hat + gloves.

Evening — semiformal. Afternoon or dinner suit or dress (suitable fabrics — silk, taffeta, velvet, soft wool, brocade, satin or lace; in spring, organza, cotton, organdy); + coat, jacket or stole (fur or fabric) + dress shoes + hose + cocktail hat + long or short gloves.

Evening — formal. Short, long or ballerina-length dress (faille, taffeta, brocade, satin, lace, tulle, net, organdy); + formal coat (taffeta, brocade, satin, fur) or stole + evening footwear.

*Certain colleges have specific clothes regulations and certain regional colleges wear regional clothes. Fabrics vary with climate and semester.

CONCERTS

Indoor. Evening: Afternoon dress or ensemble, short dinner dress, or cocktail suit; + wrap (fur or fabric) + gloves. Dinner hat optional.

Matinee: Dressmaker suit, or tailored suit, or afternoon dress or ensemble; + gloves. Hat optional.

Outdoor. Opening night: Informal evening wear + wrap or stole for evening sweater. Other evenings: Afternoon dress, short dinner dress, dressmaker suit or sport suit, sport dress; + sweater, jacket or wrap + comfortable shoes if you must walk a long distance + gloves.

CROQUET

Shorts, pedal pushers, pants or action skirt with shirt or sweater; + Oxfords, loafers or tennis shoes + bobby socks.

DANCING

Nightclub, Café or Hotel. Short dinner dress, afternoon dress, or cocktail dress; + gloves + wrap + dress shoes. Cocktail or dinner hat optional.

Public Ballroom. Evening or afternoon separates, afternoon dress, or cocktail dress; + suitable shoes + wrap. Gloves optional.

Country Club. Summer: Informal dinner dress (sheer, chiffon, lace, linen), afternoon dress, separates, or silk sport dress; + evening sweater or light wrap. Winter: Formal or informal, depending on invitation. Informal: Short dinner dress, cocktail dress, separates or afternoon dress, + dress shoes. Formal: See EVENING DRESS.

Home. Informal (following hostess's suggestion) — short dinner dress, afternoon dress, evening separates or sport dress, + suitable shoes.

DEBUTS

Debutante. Traditional debutante gown, long formal (net, lace, satin, faille — usually white but pastels permissible); + white gloves + matching shoes + simple jewelry (preferably pearls) + flowers.

Mother of Debutante. Formal evening gown, any color but black or white; + evening shoes + gloves.

Guests. Formal evening gown; + evening shoes + wrap + gloves.

DESERT RESORT

See VACATIONS

DINNERS

CITY—FORMAL

At Home. Hostess: Short or long dinner dress. Guests: Short or long dinner dress (depending on hostess's request); + evening shoes + wrap + gloves.

Restaurant, Hotel or Café (usually a dinner dance or dinner preceding other formal function). Hostess and Guests: Long or short formal dress; + evening shoes + gloves + wrap.

CITY—INFORMAL

At Home. Hostess: Afternoon dress, short dinner dress, hostess gown, or evening separates (dinner pajamas, or dinner skirt or slacks with evening sweater or blouse). Guests: afternoon dress, ensemble, or evening separates (skirt + sweater or blouse) + suitable shoes, gloves optional.

COUNTRY CLUB—FORMAL

Hostess and Guests: Short, ballerina, or full-length formal dress; + stole or evening wrap + evening shoes + gloves.

COUNTRY—INFORMAL

At Home. Hostess: Sport dress, afternoon dress, or cocktail dress, + suitable shoes. Guests: according to request of hostess.

Country Club. Sport dress, short dinner dress, afternoon dress, or separates; + suitable shoes + wrap + gloves.

DOG RACING

Spectator sport clothes — sport dress, or sport suit, or skirt with blouse or sweater; + jacket or cardigan + sport shoes + gloves. Hat optional.

DOG SHOWS

HANDLERS

Obedience. Straight skirt + blouse or sweater, or one-piece golf dress with fairly straight skirt (stripes will help make you visible to your dog — avoid green or colors with a similar tone which your dog could confuse with background greenery); + walking shoes.

Breed (where kneeling is necessary). Full-skirted shirtwaist dress, or slacks or full skirt + blouse or sweater; + walking shoes.

Field Trials. Wool slacks or safari-type pants; + sweater + windbreaker jacket + cap with earflaps + wool socks + 5-/or 9-inch boots.

SPECTATOR

Spectator sport clothes — sport or day suit, or sport or day dress, or skirt + blouse or sweater + jacket or cardigan; + sport shoes + gloves. Hat optional.

ENGAGEMENT PARTIES

See LUNCHEONS, TEAS, DINNERS

EVENING DRESS

Formal. If escort wears dinner jacket, wear short or long dinner dress, dinner suit, or evening dress; + gloves. If escort wears full dress (white tie and tails), wear formal evening gown + evening gloves.*

Informal. If escort wears street clothes, wear afternoon dress, dressmaker suit, or cocktail dress or suit, + gloves. Hat optional. If he wears dark suit, wear cocktail dress or suit, or short dinner dress; + gloves. Hat optional.

*Formality in women's dress should conform to the clothes of her escort.

FISHING

Fly Fishing. Water-repellent pants (of pima cotton if the weather is warm, safari-type cloth if cooler), with knitted cuff if you're wearing boots; + matching jacket with action sleeve (knitted cuffs a good idea) + fisherman's hat + wool socks + rubber hip-boots.

Stream Fishing. Add rubber hip-boots.

Deep Stream Fishing. Add armpit waders, chest-high and felt-soled wading shoes.

Surf fishing. Shorts or bathing suit + jacket or windbreaker + cap or hat for protection from sun.

Deep Sea Fishing. Blue jeans, denims or other sport pants + T-shirt or shirt + jacket or sweater + cap with visor or brimmed hat + rubber-soled shoes. Additional windbreaker or coat.

FOOTBALL

Sport suit, sweater and skirt, or sport dress; + topcoat + comfortable shoes + sport hat + gloves. In cool climate, or for night games, be sure the gloves are warm; add a warm scarf and warm head covering. In colder climates, add fur-trimmed, fur-lined or fur coats + galoshes or stadium boots.

FORMAL CLOTHES

See EVENING DRESS

FUNERALS

Members of the Family. Black suit or dress and coat + black hat + black gloves + black shoes. Hose need not be black, but should be dark. Veils optional. Children should be dressed preferably in white, no bright colors.

Others attending. Dark street clothes + dark hat + dark gloves + dark shoes.

GARDENING

Jeans or slacks (of any durable, washable fabric), shorts, or action skirt; + shirt or T-shirt or wash sweater + comfortable shoes + gardening gloves + hat for protection from sun. Gardening aprons with pockets for tools are useful. Suitable fabrics: Denim, cotton or wash material.

GARDEN PARTIES

Formal. Hostess: Summer afternoon or cocktail dress (light color or print). Guests: Summer afternoon dress, ensemble or cocktail dress (light color or print); + dress shoes + hat + gloves.

Informal. Hostess: Sport or summer afternoon dress, light color or print. Guests: Sport dress, summer afternoon dress or ensemble, light color or print + afternoon shoes. Hat and gloves correct but optional.

GOLF

ACTIVE

Golf dress with flared skirt or inverted pleat for action, or separate skirt, similarly made, or wraparound; + shirt, sweater + golf hat with bill + short wool golf socks + cleated golf shoes. Suitable fabrics: Cotton, thin wool or tweed. Tailored shorts permissible *on some courses only.*

Sport suit or skirt with sweater or blouse; + jacket or cardigan (windbreaker if needed) + rubber-soled or stout walking shoes. Hat and gloves optional for protection from sun.

GRADUATION

Morning. Suit, street dress, or ensemble; + street shoes + hat + gloves.

Afternoon. Dressmaker suit, afternoon dress, or ensemble; + street shoes + hat + gloves.

Evening. Afternoon dress, dressmaker suit, or dressy ensemble; + dress shoes + gloves. Hat optional.

GYM

Shorts with T-shirt or tailored cotton blouse (short-sleeved or sleeveless); + cotton anklets + tennis shoes. In weight-reducing classes, leotard and/or sweatshirt and pants can be used.

HIGH SCHOOL*

Classroom. Casual sport clothes — sweater or blouse, + skirt or jumper dress, or shirtmaker dress or sport dress; + socks + saddle shoes or loafers.

After School. Play clothes — blue jeans, denims, pants, or shorts; + sweater, T-shirt, or sport shirt, + sport or play shoes.

Evening. Sport dress, afternoon dress, or separates. For proms or formal dance: Short evening dress + coat, stole or evening sweater + suitable evening shoes + gloves.

*High school clothes are similar in fabric and line to college clothes, with these exceptions: No pants are worn on high school campuses, heels are worn only for formal and semiformal occasions, stockings are seldom worn, full skirts are more popular than sheaths for date wear, and sport clothes are worn more frequently at night.

HIKING

Shorts, pants (weight depending on weather) + wash or flannel shirt + sweater or jacket + 5 or 9 inch boots (depending on terrain and protection needed) + wool socks + visor cap (with ear-flaps if weather is cold + canvas knapsack with shoulder straps.

HORSE RACES

Sport suit, sport dress, or skirt + sweater or blouse; + jacket + sport shoes. Hat and gloves optional. Or dressmaker suit or simple afternoon ensemble, + street shoes + hat + gloves. Suitable fabrics: linen, cotton, silk, wool, tweed, depending on the weather.

HORSE SHOWS

ACTIVE

Saddle Horse Seat. Afternoon: English riding suit (any color but black) or Jodhpurs (white or beige) + contrasting coat, plain color. Night: Formal black suit.

3-Gaited Class. Formal black suit with satin lapels + white shirt with stiff collar and bow tie + black boots + top hat. *Or* white coat + black Kentucky jodhpurs + black jodhpur boots. Gloves optional and boutonnière optional.

Jumping Events. Jodhpur breeches and boots or English breeches and high English boots (breeches canary, tan or beige) + tweed or salt sack or beige jacket.

5-Gaited Class. English riding suit + soft derby + four-in-hand tie + jodhpur boots + boutonnière.

SPECTATOR

Opening Night and Closing Night. Short dinner dress, dinner suit, or cocktail suit; + wrap (fur or fabric) + cocktail or dinner hat + gloves. (Unless formal opening is announced, in which case *see* EVENING DRESS.)

Other Nights or Afternoon Performance. Spectator sports clothes, dressmaker suit, or tailored suit; + comfortable shoes. Hat and gloves optional.

HOUSEWORK

Housedress, smock, duster, or skirt or pants of any becoming length with shirt or T-shirt or wash sweater (all clothes in this category must be functional and washable, but colors can be gay); + apron suitable for work in hand — rubber, plastic, or cotton + low-heeled ties, moccasins or flats — *not* bedroom slippers.

HUNTING

Upland Game Shooting (quail, pheasant, dove). Water-repellent, safari-type pants, or down-filled pants with down-filled jacket (depending on climate); + visor cap with earlaps + leather mittens (with turn-back flap to free hand for shooting) + 9-inch boots + insulated socks + insulated underwear. In hunting quail and pheasant, wear a bright-colored, red or yellow, jacket or cap to make you visible to other hunters. In hunting dove, keep to neutral color.

Duck Hunting. Water-repellent safari-type pants and down-filled jacket, in neutral tan; + ski underwear (cotton inside, wool outside) + rubber hip-boots + beak cap.

Deer Hunting. Down-lined coat with mouton collar + visor cap with mouton earflaps + insulated rubber pac boots, 12-inch for bitter weather + insulated underwear. Wear a bright color in your jacket, red or yellow (some states specify red).

ICE HOCKEY

Warm sport clothes — sport suit, dressmaker suit, sheer wool dress, or skirt and sweater; + topcoat or fur wrap + street shoes + gloves. Hat optional. If it is very cold, add warm scarf, stadium boots.

ICE SHOWS

Opening Night. As a rule, strictly formal (*See* EVENING DRESS). Add warm wrap (fur or fabric).

Other Nights. Dressmaker suit, ensemble, afternoon dress, short dinner dress, cocktail suit, or dressy sport suit; + dress shoes + warm wrap + gloves. Hat optional.

ICE SKATING

If you skate well: short circular or pleated skirt with skating tights and sweater, cardigan or warm pullover blouse; + lined jacket + warm gloves and cap. If you wish to be more conservative: Slacks or ski pants in wool fabric treated to resist wind and water, and sweater, cardigan or pullover jersey blouse; + tight warm jacket + wool socks + warm gloves and cap.

LUNCHEONS

CITY

At Home. Hostess: Simple afternoon dress, or day dress. Guests: Dressmaker suit, simple afternoon dress, day dress, or ensemble + afternoon shoes. Hat and gloves correct but optional.

At Club or Restaurant. Hostess and Guests: Dressmaker suit, afternoon dress, or ensemble; + day shoes + hat + gloves.

COUNTRY

At Home. Hostess: Sport dress, simple afternoon dress, or skirt + sweater or blouse + day shoes. Guests: Sport dress, skirt + blouse or sweater, simple afternoon dress, or ensemble; + day shoes. Gloves and hat optional.

Outdoor or Buffet. Hostess and Guests: Sport dress, patio dress or sun dress, cotton separates + sport shoes or patio shoes.

MARKETING

CITY

Sport suit, day dress (not housedress), dress with jacket, or skirt with sweater or blouse and jacket; + coat if needed + street shoes. Hat and gloves optional.

COUNTRY

Sport clothes — Wash dress or slacks (if becoming) or skirt with sweater or blouse; + jacket or coat if needed + street or sport shoes.

MATERNITY*

Daytime. Separates (slim "window" skirts and tops), one-piece dress with adjustable waistbands, redingote, wraparound dress, jumper, duster, or maternity suit with butcher boy or boxy jacket; + low or medium-heeled shoes + gloves. Hat optional.

Evening. Slim maternity skirt, long or short, with evening top sleeveless or low-necked, or one-piece dress — flaring, gathered, pleated, or Empire waist; + evening shoes + gloves.

Casual or Sport. Slacks, Bermudas, pedal pushers or shorts + pullover top, middy, short smock or long sport shirt (worn outside pants); + sandals or sport shoes.

*Preferably maternity clothes should be solid color or small print; trim; concentrated at neckline. Hats important as eye-catchers. Basis of maternity wardrobe: Slim maternity skirt + matching or alternate tops can vary from tailored to evening look, from day fabric to evening fabric.

MOTION PICTURES

Première. Short or long evening dress, or dinner suit; + evening shoes + wrap (fur or fabric) + gloves.

Other Evenings. Day or afternoon dress, or suit (dressmaker, tailored or sport); + dress shoes + wrap as needed. Gloves optional.

Daytime. Day dress, suit, or spectator sport clothes; + street shoes. Gloves and hat optional.

MOUNTAIN CLIMBING

Sweater or shirt with heavy pants or corduroy knickers; + hooded parka + 6-inch moccasin-type boots (with rubber cleats) + heavy socks + leather gloves.

MOUNTAIN RESORTS

See VACATIONS

OPEN HOUSE

Day. Dressmaker suit, afternoon dress, ensemble, cocktail dress, or suit; + dress shoes + hat and gloves.

Evening. Cocktail dress or suit, dinner dress or suit, or informal evening dress; + evening shoes + gloves. Evening hat optional. Hostess will indicate degree of formality.

OPERA

Opening Night. Usually formal. (*See* EVENING DRESS).

Outdoor Opening Night. Informal summer evening dress; + evening shoes + wrap, stole or evening sweater.

Other Evenings. Dinner suit, dinner dress, cocktail suit, or dark afternoon dress; + dress shoes + gloves + dinner or cocktail hat (optional) + wrap. Furs suitable.

Matinees. Afternoon dress, or dressmaker suit; + hat + gloves + street shoes.

Other Evenings. Afternoon dress, short dinner dress, dressmaker suit, or ensemble; + wrap, sweater or jacket; + comfortable shoes + gloves.

PICNIC

Casual clothes — blue jeans, slacks, or shorts, with sport shirt; + cardigan sweater or jacket; + sneakers or moccasins. Or sport dress or skirt and blouse; + jacket or sweater; + sport shoes, sandals or flats. Straw play hat optional.

PING-PONG

Any length slacks or shorts with action blouse or sweater; or active sport dress; + flats or tennis shoes.

PLANE TRAVEL

See TRAVEL

PLAYGROUND

When you take your children to the playground: Sport dress (with easy skirt), sport suit, simple day dress, skirt and sweater or blouse; + jacket. Or slacks with blouse and jacket. Comfortable shoes and large purse (to carry all the extras). Play hat optional.

PRIZE FIGHTS

Suit, dress, ensemble, or spectator sport clothes — sport dress, sport suit; + street shoes. Hat and gloves optional. Coat in cool weather.

RAINWEAR

Matching rainwear can turn a rainy day into a gay one: water-repellent coat (fabric or plastic), hooded or with matching cap or water-repellent scarf. Or hooded car coat + gloves + boots (plastic or rubber) + umbrella.

RECEPTIONS*

See also CHRISTENINGS, DEBUTS, WEDDINGS

Afternoon. Formal afternoon dress or ensemble; + dress shoes + hat + gloves.

Evening. Long or short evening dress + evening shoes + gloves.

*For receptions following any function, dress as if you had attended that function.

RIDING

English Park Riding (bridal path). Jodhpur breeches (beige or white) with tailored shirt or Tattersall; + tweed coat or salt sack coat or linen coat + jodhpur boots (black or tan) + soft hat (black or tan). Or English high boots (black or tan) + breeches (black or brown). There are two kinds of jodhpur breeches: park pants, without peg and without cuff; and Kentucky jodhpurs (regular jods), with peg and cuff. Either are correct.

Western Riding. Blue jeans or frontier pants with Western snap-button shirt; + frontier jacket + Western boots + chaps (for the range) + Western belt + cowboy hat (felt or straw, depending on the weather). Tie optional.

Western Parade Riding. Matching outfit, jacket and pants in any material you choose, from gabardine to leather decorated in sequins or fringe — simple black leather very high-style + frontier hat + Western boots + gauntlet gloves + tie.

For the Hunt. This is very formal — canary-colored breeches obligatory (jodhpurs never); + black Melton hunt coat + high black boots with patent-leather cuffs obligatory + white shirt + stock tie + cork-lined derby or black velvet hunt cap + buckskin gloves.

ROLLERSKATING

Action skirt, or slacks, with blouse or sweater; + wool socks + cardigan sweater or jacket.

SAFARI

Select clothes not for warmth but for durability. Shorts of light-weight Supima cotton, + pants of water-repellent safari-type cloth, with cotton blouse; + belted bush coat + water-repellent jacket for bad weather + desert boots (for jeep travel) + 5-inch hiking boots or 9-inch moccasin boots (depending on how much walking you'll do in the rough).

SHOPPING

CITY

Suit, street dress, or dress with jacket or coat; + street shoes + hat + gloves (color and weight depend on time of year).

COUNTRY

Shirtmaker dress, sport dress, or skirt, with sweater or blouse; + street shoes. Hat and gloves optional.

SHOWERS

Morning or Luncheon. Day dress, dressmaker suit, ensemble, or dressy sport dress; + afternoon shoes + hat + gloves.

Tea or Cocktail. Afternoon dress, cocktail dress, or cocktail suit; + dress shoes + cocktail hat + gloves.

Evening. Short dinner dress, dinner suit, cocktail dress, or suit; + dress shoes + gloves. Evening hat optional.

SKEET AND TRAP SHOOTING

Slacks, frontier trousers, or shorts, with shirt or sweater; + silhouette shooting-vest or sweater (royal blue for skeet shooting; maroon for trap shooting) + visored cap + cotton or wool socks + ankle-height shoes, jodhpur or chukker boots, or walking Oxfords. (Out West: Western boots and frontier pants.)

SKIING

Ski pants of water-repellent stretch material (light colors smartest) with ski parka (hood attached) and pullover ski sweater or wool shirt to wear under parka; + candy-striped ski underwear (cotton inside, wool outside) + wool socks + ski boots + mittens and over-mittens + hip pouch to wear on belt (of fur or to match ski pants).

After-ski Activities. After-ski pants of stretch material in multi-color stripes or prints + after-ski hip-length jacket or one-piece after-ski suit of stretch material + hip pouch + after-ski boots, lambswool lined + wool socks.

SKIN-DIVING

Bathing suit (warm or shallow water). Or frog-man suit (winter or deep water) + goggles + mask + flippers + weighted belt + cap (optional).

SNOW-WEAR

Heavy inner-lined coat (preferably of water-repellent fabric) or full-length hooded car coat (if coat has no hood, add cap, scarf, or hood); + gloves or mittens (wool or leather innerlined) + muffler (wool) + snowboots (fleece-lined) or galoshes.

SPORTS CAR RACING

Shirt or sweater and pants, shorts, or heavy cotton overalls; + hooded sweater or parka + sport shoes (loafers) + bobby socks + leather gloves + crash helmet + racing goggles.

SWIMMING

For good figure: Two-piece or one-piece swimsuit. For mature figure: Dressmaker suit, with skirt. Beachcoat (terrycloth or water-absorbent fabric), cape, towel or poncho; + sandals, thong or rope-soled footwear + bathing cap. *Bathing suit should be worn only in bathing area.*

TEAS

CITY

At Home. Hostess: Afternoon dress, or dressy separates. Guests: Dressmaker suit, afternoon dress, or ensemble; + afternoon shoes + hat + gloves.

At Club or Restaurant. Hostess and Guests: Dressmaker suit, afternoon dress, cocktail dress or suit, or ensemble; + dress shoes + hat + gloves.

COUNTRY

At Home. Hostess and Guests: Dressy spectator sport clothes or afternoon dress + suitable shoes. For guests: hat and gloves.

TENNIS

ACTIVE

White, is imperative. Shorts + T-shirt or blouse. Or one-piece sleeveless dress with flared skirt. Or shift dress (loose belt, short pleated skirt). Or short culottes + overblouse. Wool socks + tennis shoes. Hat with bill optional.

SPECTATOR

Sport dress, sport suit or skirt with blouse or sweater, or simple day dress; + sport shoes + hat for protection from sun + gloves. Suitable fabrics: Linen, cotton, print, sport silk in light colors.

THEATER

Opening Night. Long or short evening clothes. (*See* EVENING DRESS)

Other Evenings. Short dinner dress, dinner suit, cocktail dress, cocktail suit, dressmaker suit, or afternoon dress (dark costume preferable); + dress shoes + stole or wrap (furs suitable) + gloves. Hat, if worn, should be small.

Matinees. Afternoon dress, dressmaker suit, or tailored suit; + afternoon shoes + gloves. Hat, if worn, should be small.

Summer Theater. Informal summer day or dinner clothes; + dress shoes + sweater or stole + gloves.

TOBOGGANING

See SKIING

TRACK MEETS

Casual clothes — sport suit, sport dress, simple day dress, or skirt and sweater; + sport shoes + hat and gloves as protection from sun. For night meets, add heavy sweater or coat. Hat purely optional; in brisk weather, a knitted cap or scarf.

TRAIN

See TRAVEL

TRAVEL

BOAT

To Board. Suit, tailored dress, sport dress, or sport suit; + topcoat + street shoes + hat + gloves + good-sized purse for passport, etc.

On Deck. Casual clothes during the day — shirtmaker dress, slacks or skirt and sweater or blouse; + jacket or coat + sport or play shoes. Hat optional.

For Active Sports. Bathing suit + terrycloth coat (or other bathing robe), or sunsuit, or shorts + T-shirt or blouse; + playshoes.

For Dinner. On big liners first night out, wear day clothes. Other evenings, dinner dress, evening separates + evening shoes + stole or short wrap of fabric or light fur.

For Cruise Trip. More casual look, cotton and sun dresses for deck wear, summer dinner dresses.

BUS

Sport dress, sport suit, or skirt (easy for sitting) and blouse or sweater; + comfortable shoes + hat + gloves + good-sized purse. Tailored slacks are acceptable for long trips.

PLANE

To Board. Dress with jacket or suit of crease-resistant fabric (two-piece costume best, jacket can be removed, sweater can be added, dark or medium colors preferable); + street shoes + hat + bag + gloves. Since weight of luggage must be kept at minimum, carry coat or raincoat and make-up case or overnight bag with drugs, make-up, folding slippers, sweater or additional skirt and blouse.

For Long Air Trip. Carry extra skirt or slacks + extra blouse + slippers or flats.

TRAIN

To Board. Suit, sport dress, sport suit, tailored dress, or ensemble (in dark or medium color); + topcoat or raincoat + small hat + street shoes + bag + gloves.

For Overnight Trip. Add tailored dressing gown, nightgown or pajamas + slippers + bag for toilet articles.

For Long Trip. Add extra sport dress + blouse and skirt + tailored slacks if becoming + sweater + comfortable shoes.

TROUSSEAU*

Going Away. Dress, or suit; + hat + gloves + coat. Sport dress, afternoon dress, dinner or cocktail dress, evening wrap, coat or stole + matching accessories with each.

Lingerie. Bridal nightdress with matching negligee + other night-dresses or pajamas + sleepcoat or robe + slips, half-slips + girdles, brassières, panties, etc. + bedroom slippers.

*Clothes for trousseau determined by locale of honeymoon — weight and color of fabric to suit season and weather + sport and recreational clothes needed for sports activities. (*See* VACATIONS.)

VACATIONS

CITY

Sight-seeing. Sport suit, tailored suit, day dress, or sport dress; + jacket or coat, depending on the weather, + comfortable walking shoes + gloves. Hat optional.

In foreign cities, never wear shorts or tight slacks in public.

If you are going to be gone all day, better wear the hat and carry an extra pair of fresh gloves in your purse, then you're prepared for luncheon anywhere.

Evening Activities. See COCKTAIL PARTIES, DINNER, THEATER, OPERA, CONCERTS, SHOPPING, SHOWS. In large cities, black or dark colors preferable.

BEACH RESORT

Daytime. Sport dress or slacks or shorts, the length becoming to you, or sun dress, skirt + blouse or halter + jacket or sweater + sport shoes or sandals.

Active Sports. See BOATING, FISHING, SWIMMING, BEACH. It is important to wear beach shoes with swimming or beach wear. If you can't wear flats, wear sport or beach shoes with wedges.

Evening. Summer afternoon or sport dress. (For formal evenings, chiffon, organdy or cotton informal dinner dress + evening shoes + evening sweater or stole.)

DESERT RESORT

Daytime. Desert wear is very casual — wash dress, denims, sunsuit, shorts + shirt or halter, + cool, comfortable sandals + straw hat for protection from sun.

Active Sports. See RIDING (Western), SWIMMING, TENNIS, GOLF.

Evening. Sport, afternoon or simple dinner dress, cotton or print + suitable shoes. For more formal occasion, sheer or cotton summer informal evening dress + evening shoes + evening sweater or stole. The desert gets cool at night.

MOUNTAIN RESORT

Daytime. Sport suit, sport dress, slacks, blue jeans or denims, skirt + sweater or blouse + jacket + walking shoes or boots + topcoat or raincoat.

Active Sports. See RIDING (WESTERN), HIKING, MOUNTAIN CLIMBING, SWIMMING.

Evening. Sport dress and matching sweater, or simple dinner dress; + suitable shoes + wrap or evening sweater. Add warm coat (fur or fabric) for cooler weather.

WATER SKIING

Action swim suit + swim cap. To wear when you're through: terrycloth coat or cotton fabric coat + thongs, rope-soled beach shoes or (if you can't wear flats) beach sandals with cork wedge.

WEDDINGS*

FORMAL DAYTIME

Bride. Bridal gown, full-length, with or without train. White or ivory preferable, pastels acceptable. Satin, lace, chiffon, net, faille, brocade, peau de soie. In summer, organdy or sheer cotton. Neckline moderate, not too bare. Long sleeves preferable — if very short, use long gloves (rip ring finger for ceremony). Veil (full-length or fingertip) lace, net or tulle. Fabric shoes to match dress. Bouquet and/or prayerbook. Pearls are the proper jewelry.

Bridesmaids. Bridesmaids' gowns full-length to match bridal gown and in similar style (Empire, Victorian, etc.). All may wear the same color, shades of the same color, or pairs of different colors. Hats or headdresses may match or contrast with gown. Hat, shoes and gloves may match. Bouquet, or sheaf of flowers.

*For weddings in church, it is customary that all women, bridal party and guests, wear some head-covering; in some churches it is obligatory. Arms should be covered, gloves are correct.

Matron or Maid of Honor. Gown of formal length to match bridal gown and in similar style as bridesmaids' gowns but different color, or in same color as bridesmaids but different style; + hat or headdress to match or contrast with gown. Hat, shoes and gloves may match. Bouquet, or sheaf of flowers.

Flower Girl. Dress may match bridesmaids in color, but fabric should be youthful (nylon, organdy) + flowers or other head-covering. Carries flowers or petals.

Ring-bearer. If girl, dresses the same as the flower girl, but carries ring fastened to small pillow.

Mother of the Bride; Mother of the Groom. Afternoon dress of silk, faille, lace, or taffeta — in gray, beige, pastel, or medium tones — dressmaker silk suit or ensemble acceptable; + hat + gloves and shoes matching each other and matching or contrasting with costume. Black or white not used in dress or accessories. Corsage.

Wedding Guests. Street-length afternoon dresses, silk suits, or ensembles; + afternoon shoes + hats + gloves. (Guests do not wear flowers.)

FORMAL EVENING

Bride. Bridal gown, full-length with sweep or train. White or ivory preferable. Satin, lace, brocade, tulle, peau de soie, velvet can be used in winter. Neckline not too bare. Long sleeves preferable; if very short, use long gloves (rip ring finger for ceremony). Medium or full-length veil, usually with head-dress and of lace, net or tulle; + fabric shoes to match dress + bouquet and/or prayerbook. Pearls are the proper jewelry.

Bridesmaids. See WEDDING, FORMAL DAYTIME.

Matron or Maid of Honor. See WEDDING, FORMAL DAYTIME.

Flower Girl. See WEDDING, FORMAL DAYTIME.

Ring-bearer. See WEDDING, FORMAL DAYTIME.

Mother of the Bride; Mother of the Groom. Dinner dress of lace, chiffon, silk or faille in beige, gray or soft pastel color + hat or head-covering + dress shoes and gloves same color as dress or contrasting. (Black or white not used in dress or accessories.) Carry corsage of flowers.

Wedding Guests. Dinner dresses; + dinner hats + dress shoes + gloves. Guests do not wear flowers.

INFORMAL DAYTIME

Bride. Ballerina-length dress and short veil, or street-length dress (white, ivory or light color preferable) with hat or headdress and face veil (optional); + shoes + gloves to match. Or dressmaker suit (in any color except black) + hat + shoes + gloves to match. Small bouquet or corsage.

Bridesmaids. Dresses of same length as bride's dress, in pastel color (since informal weddings have fewer bridesmaids, usually all one color); + hat or headdress + matching or contrasting gloves and shoes. If bride wears dressmaker suit, so will bridesmaids. Flowers.

Matron of Honor. Dress of same length and style as bride + hat or headdress + matching or contrasting shoes and gloves. If bride wears dressmaker suit, so will matron. Flowers.

Mother of the Bride; Mother of the Groom. Afternoon or day dress, any color except black or white + afternoon shoes. Head-covering and gloves preferable in church, optional at home. Corsage.

Wedding Guests. Day or afternoon dresses + afternoon shoes. Gloves and hats preferable for church, optional at home. No flowers.

INFORMAL EVENING

Bride. Long or short dinner dress (white, ivory or pastel) + headdress with or without veil + shoes to match dress + gloves if arms are bare (the covered-up look is preferable) + flowers or corsage. With street-length dress, headdress of flowers or short veil may be used.

Bridesmaids. Length and style of dresses conform with that of bride, in pastel color. Since informal weddings have fewer bridesmaids, usually all one color + matching shoes + head-covering (in church) + gloves. Flowers.

Maid or Matron of Honor. Dress may be same style as bridesmaids but different color, or same color as bridesmaids but different style; + matching shoes + head-covering (in church) + gloves. Flowers.

Mother of the Bride; Mother of the Groom. Long or short dinner dress to conform with bride. Beige, gray or pastel (no black, no white) + suitable shoes + hat and gloves if in church. Corsage.

Wedding Guests. Dinner dresses of same length and formality as those of bride and wedding party; + dress shoes + hats and gloves if in church. No flowers.

CIVIL SERVICE MARRIAGE

Bride. Street-length dress, or suit (any color except black) + hat with small face veil if desired + day shoes + gloves (carried, not worn at ceremony) + corsage.

Attendants. Dress in keeping with bride.

DOUBLE WEDDING

Brides. May or may not dress alike.
Attendants. Harmonize with bride.

GARDEN WEDDING*

Bride — Formal or Informal. Usually wears bridal dress of summer fabric (organdy, lace, embroidered sheer, cotton); + flower headdress with or without veil + gloves or mitts + prayerbook or bouquet + matching shoes.

*In garden weddings, the whole effect is more simple. Many times, garden flowers are used for bride instead of traditional bridal bouquet.

Attendants. Length and style conform to dress of bride, pastel colors (summer fabric). Garden hats or flower headdresses; + matching gloves or mitts + matching footwear + flowers.

Mother of the Bride; Mother of the Groom. Summer dress, street-length or long, pastel color (chiffon, crepe or lace); + hat + gloves + matching shoes + corsage.

Guests. Afternoon dresses, long or short, soft prints (lace, crepe, chiffon); + hat + gloves + shoes to match. Guests do not wear flowers.

OLDER BRIDE

Bride. May wear wedding gown, but afternoon costume preferable. Can be white, but pastel color more usual. If veil is used, should be short. With afternoon gown, hat or head-covering + matching gloves + matching footwear + flowers, worn or carried.
Attendants. Costumes and accessories conform to bride's.

RECTORY WEDDING

Bride. Street dress, suit, ensemble (any color except black). Hat with veil (not wedding veil). Matching shoes + matching gloves + flowers worn or carried.

Attendants. Costume and accessories conform to bride.

SECOND MARRIAGE

Bride. Suit or simple dress, pastel (any color except black or white). Hat or headdress, with face veil optional; + matching shoes + matching gloves + flowers worn.

Attendants. Costume and accessories conform to bride's.

Guests. Suits, ensembles, day dresses + suitable shoes + hats + gloves. Guests do not wear flowers.

WRESTLING MATCHES

See PRIZE FIGHTS